W9-BTJ-867

# Stress and Tension Control

# Stress and Tension Control

Edited by

F. J. McGuigan

University of Louisville
Louisville, Kentucky

Wesley E. Sime

University of Nebraska
Lincoln, Nebraska

and

J. Macdonald Wallace

West London Institute of Higher Education
London, England



PLENUM PRESS · NEW YORK AND LONDON

Library of Congress Cataloging in Publication Data

International Interdisciplinary Conference on Stress and Tension Control, London. 1979.
Stress and tension control.
Proceedings of the International Interdisciplinary Conference on Stress and Tension Control held in London, Sept. 10–14, 1979, and sponsored by the American Association for the Advancement of Tension Control and the West London Institute of Higher Education.
Includes index.
1. Stress (Physiology)–Congresses. 2. Stress (Psychology)–Congresses. 3. Relaxation–Congresses. 4. Medicine, Psychosomatic–Congresses. I. McGuigan, Frank J. II. Sime, Wesley E. III. Wallace, J. Macdonald. IV. American Association for the Advancement of Tension Control. V. West London Institute of Higher Education. VI. Title. [DNLM: 1. Relaxation–Congresses. 2. Stress, Psychological–Prevention and control–Congresses. WM172 I51s 1979]
BF575.S75I57 1979 616'.001'9 80-16444
ISBN 0-306-40450-8

Sponsored by
The American Association for the Advancement of Tension Control
and
The West London Institute of Higher Education

Proceedings of the International Interdisciplinary Conference on Stress and Tension Control, held in London, England, September 10–14, 1979.


A Division of Plenum Publishing Corporation
227 West 17th Street, New York, N.Y. 10011



Printed in the United States of America

# IN MEMORIAM

We wish to dedicate these proceedings to the memory of W. Horsley Gantt, M.D., a great scientist who died February 26, 1980, at age 87, after a life of service to humanity. The recipient of many honors for his work in developing theories concerning neurosis, Schizokinesis, and Autokinesis, Dr. Gantt was a physiologist, psychiatrist, and a true scientist in every noble meaning of the word. He was president of the American Association for the Advancement of Tension Control during the last year of his active and productive life, and spoke at the London Conference, of which these proceedings are the result. Dr. Gantt will be sorely missed by all who knew him and his exceptional abilities as a seeker of knowledge.

# PREFACE

"Tension" is an internationally recognized word. Its omnipresence in our public media--in our newspapers, on TV, in magazines, and on radio--as well as in our everyday conversations indicate that we are well aware of the problems of over-tenseness. Pulp newspapers and magazines increase their sales with promises of quick relief for tension problems. Business executives complain at the end of the day of being "uptight", and often accept a hotel chain's invitation to "unwind" at their bar. Soap operas attract large audiences, in part capitalizing on tension problems--irritable arguments between husband and wife seem interminable!

Indeed, the entire world is aware of the need to control tensions. Such widespread needs invite varied "solutions", with the most attractive appearing ones offering promises of quick and easy cures.

The market for tension reduction has been exploited in numerous ingenious ways for centuries but I think never more than today. People with serious tension disorders often eagerly seize promises of easy relief, regardless of cost. Those who suffer headaches, spastic colon, essential hypertension, back pains, phobias and general anxiety are especially sensitized to tension disorders and potential cures.

The American Association for the Advancement of Tension Control is dedicated to the elimination of tension problems through a two-pronged attack: through the immediate technological application of tension control principles that now exist, and by encouraging scientific research to further develop our methods. We hope to help the public to practice those technics of tension control that have sound scientific and clinical validation; this is accomplished in part through the direct and objective measurement of tension, principally through electromyography. This is because the classical, standard definition of tension is contraction of the skeletal muscle; and relaxation is the elongation of skeletal muscle fibers. The consequences of these accepted scientific definitions of tension and relaxation for prophylactic and for therapeutic purposes are enormous, as these proceedings illustrate.

To realize our long term goals of bringing effective tension control to the peoples of the world we invite the cooperation of all interested individuals. By working vigorously together our interdisciplinary efforts should bring us increasingly close to success.

F. J. McGuigan

CONTENTS

## TENSION AND LIFE



## STRESS AND CARDIOVASCULAR DISORDERS

## PAIN AND TENSION CONTROL



## TENSION IN DENTISTRY



## TENSION AND HEADACHES



## TENSION AND PSYCHIATRY

## TENSION AND ANXIETY



## TENSION AND BIOFEEDBACK



## TENSION AND STUTTERING



## PRINCIPLES AND APPLICATIONS OF TENSION CONTROL

# TENSION AND LIFE

# TENSION AND STRESS

Robert E. Rinehart, M.D.

Director, Rinehart Clinic
Portland, Oregon

Tension as referred to here, is habitual or persistent reflex contraction of voluntary muscles. This habit pattern arises through involuntary practice, because of bracing to real or imagined uncertainties and/or to painful stimuli. Stress is defined as the reaction(s) of the organism to any noxious stimulus. Therefore tension is simply one form of stress, comparable to shivering, inflammation, or any other reaction to unpleasant or harmful stimuli.

Difficulties arise because: (a.) We are continually exposed to a multitude of uncertainties resulting in frequent instinctive tightening, and (b.) Any repeated muscular action is apt to become a habit pattern. Those of us who happen to be above the average level of intelligence have excellent imaginative ability with which to conjure up uncertainties. Those of us who tend to be perfectionists are never quite certain about anything. People who possess these two characteristics are prone to develop a habit pattern of bracing and become perpetually "stressed."

Initially this habit pattern results in a feeling of exhilaration, frequently leading to physical overexertion. Later feelings of shakiness, jitteriness and uneasiness occur, followed by fatigue. For a time fatigue may be masked by exhilaration. Later fatigue becomes prominent in the morning, after sleeping tense all night. By afternoon sufficient tightening has occurred to result in masking of fatigue by exhilaration.

In time fatigued muscles begin to cramp. When this is noticed it is frequently prominent in neck and/or lower back, classicly called "tension headache" or "lumbago." Of course it is well known that many things give us a pain in the neck or a pain in the buttocks. These are favorite locations for pain of this nature because the initial tightening is in preparation for fight (tightening of neck and shoulders) or flight (tightening of hips and lower back). From this starting point of fatigue and spasm, at times modified by altered immune responses, there arises a plethora of musculoskeletal disabilities generally known as rheumatism and arthritis.

Unfortunately these untoward musculoskeletal reactions are only the beginning of a variety of disorders due to prolonged stress. Any or several of the physiopathological disorders described by Selye (1952) as the "Adaptation Syndrome" may occur, plus a variety of emotional disturbances. Prominent among these are visceral disturbances manifested by cardiovascular and gastrointestinal malfunction. They arise because of constant bombardment of cerebral control centers by proprioceptive impulses originating in tense muscles. Initially there is hyperarousal originating in stimulation of the reticular formation. Once this is initiated it causes the organism to be perpetually on guard and more sensitive to real or imaginary uncertainty. As this increased proprioceptive stimulus reaches the hypothalamus a host of visceral disturbances are manifested by flushing, sweating, chilling, upset stomach, constipation, diarrhea, palpitation, blurred vision, dry mouth, wet hands and feet, etc.

As the limbic system becomes involved in this neuronal hyperactivity emotional disturbances arise. These are manifested by feelings of irritability, apprehension and anxiety. This is the basis of and explanation for the variety of psychoneuroses which previously have been inexplicable.

Depression arises as the cerebral cortex, with its perception-association functions, becomes involved by over-stimulation. The organism can no longer associate sensory stimuli from various sources and is forced to withdraw as far as possible from any stimulation.

In view of the amount and variety of suffering arising from this one source it is no wonder that people have been seeking means to relieve tension. Unfortunately most "systems," i.e. yoga, transcendental meditation, biofeedback, autogenic training, zen, etc. for relief of tension are only transiently effective. The only practical system for general application is that of Jacobson (1938, 1964) called "progressive relaxation." This requires the services of teachers who have been trained in anatomy, physiology, kinesiology, neurology and other basic disciplines. Another system, somewhat less scientific and therefore less effective, is that of Feldenkrais (1972) described in his book "Awareness Through Movement." This system also is best learned with the help of a trained teacher.

REFERENCES

Feldenkrais, M., 1972, "Awareness Through Movement," Harper and Row, New York.
Jacobson, E., 1938, 11th impression, 1971, "Progressive Relaxation," University of Chicago Press, Chicago.
Jacobson, E., 1964, "You Must Relax," McGraw-Hill, New York.
Selye, H., 1952, "The Story of the Adaptive Syndrome," Acta Foundation, Chicago.

# AROUSAL OF THE BRAIN AND COPING MECHANISMS

Ivor H. Mills, Ph.D., M.D., F.R.C.P.

Endocrinologist, Professor of Medicine
Cambridge University
Cambridge, England

The challenges which the brain has to cope with present themselves in a variety of ways, perhaps as a poisonous snake in the grass, perhaps as the self-imposed drive to pass an important examination. In general, challenges fall into two groups (1.) those imposed from outside and (2.) those which are self-generated.

In either case, certain responses of the nervous system are similar. The information that an outside threat exists has to be perceived by one of the senses. The transmission of the nervous impulses is in part to the appropriate region of the cerebral cortex and thus to the consciousness but in part it is fed into a specialized system within the spinal cord and brain which is designed to excite the nervous system to appreciate novelty or danger. This is the reticular formation. It is developed to gather messages from all possible sources and to coordinate them in terms of the severity of threat which is imposed. Each individual message may be exaggerated or suppressed in terms of the importance of the threat. Awareness of a cat brushing past one's leg may be totally suppressed if one hears a sudden scream of terror.

The reticular formation continues into the brain from related structures in the cord. It determines various types of excitement or arousal within the nervous system. One of these is a manifestation in the electroencephalogram (EEG) which can bring about the change from relative slow waves which are synchronous and fairly high in amplitude and related to the resting or sleep state, to fast, desynchronised, low amplitude waves which are typical of arousal.

These EEG changes can be mimicked by certain drugs: atropine or other antagonists of acetyl choline produce the sleep pattern whereas drugs mimicking acetyl choline, or preventing its destruction, as physostigmine does, produce the arousal pattern.

The second type of arousal is behavioral arousal. Usually it is associated with EEG arousal but the association can be broken by means of drugs. Frightening challenges would prepare one behaviorally for action in case of need. If the challenge is sudden, unexpected and intense, it may precipitate the third type of arousal, namely, that of the autonomic nervous system. This response may be manifest as sweating, erection of the hairs in the skin and palpitations. These phenomena are especially designed for a physical response to the challenge, for attack or running out of the way of what is threatening.

However, internal challenges not infrequently produce similar arousal phenomena even though no physical response is likely to be called for. This is obvious if one is looking at a film or television picture, though the reality of the scene may make one feel that it is being experienced and the arousal responses, therefore, may seem compatible with this. On the other hand, mental challenges may produce some degree of autonomic arousal: for instance, doing mental arithmetic will cause elevation of the blood pressure (Ludbrook et al., 1975).

## AROUSAL AND EFFICIENCY

The effectiveness of the brain depends upon the degrees of arousal. If one has a vigilance task in which it is necessary to spot a relatively infrequent event, the concentration commonly flags if the events are very infrequent. The mind begins to wander and when the event occurs it goes unnoticed. This is of importance in the observation of dials in relation to processes in industry. It is now well established that arousal can be elevated by some non-distracting device, e.g. music, and then awareness of the infrequent events is likely to be more accurate.

We know from experimental studies that electrical stimulation of the reticular formation produces responses which depend upon the intensity of stimulation. Initially it produces an alerting effect or the "anticipatory set". At this stage the pulse rate slows and blood pressure is not raised though increased sweating may occur. If nothing is observed as a potential danger by the animal, it proceeds with its ordinary activity. Higher stimulation produces fear and the animal is likely to run and hide in the corner of the cage. Still higher stimulation causes chaotic, uncoordinated activity, rushing around quite aimlessly.

Figure 1 represents the increase in efficiency with stimulation of arousal. With mental activity, if arousal is driven too hard,

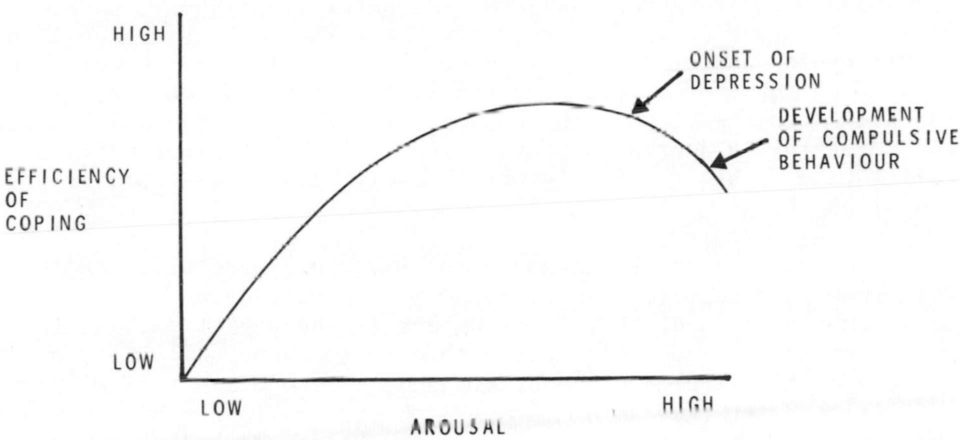


Fig. 1. Bi-phasic relationship between arousal and coping efficiency. Beyond a certain point further elevation leads to depression which may remain masked. Still further elevation of arousal leads to development of compulsive thought disorders and compulsive behavior.

efficiency reaches a plateau. In most people, they are unable to drive their arousal higher than this; fatigue sets in and they rest. However, if the person is very highly motivated, or is fired by intense ambition, arousal may be driven still further and then not only may efficiency fall but depression may then set in. Rather surprisingly, most people are not aware of the fall off in efficiency with excessive drive or arousal.

With obsessional personalities, the drive to achieve some goal may continue long after the peak of efficiency is reached. It is then that we may see the development of compulsive behavior.

## EVERYDAY LIFE

Challenges arise from outside the brain even in those who have no demanding job or competitive life to lead. If one's house is struck by lightning in a storm and structurally damaged, it demands extensive thought to work out all the steps that will be required to restore it to normal. Not the least of the challenges is the uncertainty as to whether the insurance company will consider the policy high enough in value to warrant payment of the full costs of repairs.

If, shortly afterwards, the man is told he is about to be made redundant and he knows he will have difficulty in obtaining new employment, he is faced with a whole new series of challenges with which he is forced to cope if he has a dependent family. While he is wrestling with these problems his son might have a motorcycle accident and spend weeks in a hospital: his daughter might have a sudden and unexpected break-up in a love affair. All these represent challenges to his brain, and also to other members of his family. He might well be able to cope for a while but the strain on his daughter might be too great and she becomes increasingly irritable as she loses sleep and moves into a depressed state. The irritability inevitably leads to friction within the family which itself becomes an important additional challenge.

How long can the brain go on meeting one demand after another? With some personalities the response to too many demands is to give up attempting to meet them. Opting out is one way of failing to cope, but it at least leaves the person able to go on normally with other aspects of his life. On the other hand, if the man with family responsibilities strives hard to cope with the challenges he may reach the state where he can stand no more and he enters a depressed state.

In Table 1 are shown the everyday events which may lead to excessive demands upon the coping mechanism of the brain. In their book "Social origins of depression", Professor George Brown and Dr. Tirril Harris indicate the results of their studies on the quantitation of everyday challenging events. In those who had been diagnosed as depressed the frequency of events, and especially major challenges, was appreciably higher than in the people in their control group. The time during which there had been excessive demands on coping before depression set in was frequently several months. The time scale is important. A few major events over three or four months may be more than most people can tolerate.

## INTERACTION OF EXCITING AND STRESSFUL EVENTS

For most people leisure time is thought of as a time for enjoyment when the cares of the day are cast away. However, the studies of Levi and his colleagues (1972) have shown that a variety of common types of enjoyment such as watching amusing, exciting or frightening films, will produce exactly the same rise in adrenaline excretion as is seen in invoice clerks transferred from weekly wages to piece-work rates. The increase in adrenaline excretion reflects the higher level of excitement of the brain. Only watching films of natural scenery led to a fall in adrenaline excretion.

It is known that on nights when major boxing matches are being televised there is an increase in the number of patients experiencing anginal attacks or even coronary thrombosis. This is a sphere where the relationship between leisure activity and deleterious response is obvious. It is not so obvious that all major types of excitement add up in terms of coping ability, even though some are pleasantly exciting occasions and others are traumaticly exciting. The sum of the arousing effects is what determines the ultimate response in the brain. When the total demands are too high, depression sets in.

Table 1. Events Making Demands on the Coping Mechanism

Moving house

Working for examinations

Friction in personal relationships, at home or at work

Falling in love

Broken love affair/marriage

Illicit love affair

Loss of sleep because of ill children

Mother, with young family, working "twilight" shift

Wife alone a lot because husband at sea, etc.

Severe illness in family

Accidents to house, car, etc.

Wife/husband/children battering

Baby constantly stimulated to stop it crying

Exciting films/television

Exciting sport, boxing, rock-climbing, ice-hockey

Some individuals are quite unaware of the build up of underlying depression because it may remain masked (Pollitt and Young, 1971). The process of masking the depression is brought about by the arousal level of the brain. When this is very high, appreciable depression may be generated without being obvious. The presense of the masked depression may be dramatically revealed if the arousal level of the brain is suddenly lowered. Most commonly this occurs with alcohol when more than usual has been consumed at a good party. The next morning when the man or woman wakes up intense depression may grip him and prevent the execution of, perhaps, relatively undemanding tasks.

Other ways in which depression may suddenly be un-masked are the use of antidepressant drugs or even learning transendental meditation.

Both of these may act quite quickly to lower the brain's arousal level and the person may suddenly be overcome with unexpected depression. If this occurs with antidepressant drugs, it requires an immediate increase in the dose to bring the depression under control. Sometimes the likely individuals to suffer in this way may be selected before hand: commonly they have sleep disturbance and some upset of sexual functioning, e.g. change in pattern of menstruation or loss of libido in women; impotence in men. If both these types of problem occur at the same time, meditation should be embarked upon with great caution.

Some individuals, especially teenagers, discover that if they take part in exciting things it may mask their depression and so make them feel much better. Sometimes the discovery is made by accident. This particularly applies to the current craze in young women to begin strict dieting, even when they are not overweight. The slim image has been fashionable for women since the early nineteen sixties and was epitomized by Twiggy. Often for no good reason a girl, or a group of them, goes on a diet. Initially weight loss may be slight but there often comes a time when it is excessive. The family then tries to influence her to eat more normally. It may take a great deal of persuasion but when she does eat more, she realizes that she does not feel so lively and she has to make more effort to do her work. At this point she may well return to her strict diet because she has discovered what Benedict described in 1915 in professional fasters. Starvation produces mental stimulation and a sense of elation; the brain is more excited and can cope better with problems; it works faster and more accurately with less sense of fatigue.

This response to self-starvation is particularly going to benefit the girl studying for examinations. Indeed 75% of young women with anorexia nervosa start dieting in the year they are studying for an important examination. Once they have realized the effect of strict dieting on arousal level, they are very difficult to dissuade from their self-starvation.

Although students commonly work into the night to do their work, a few find out that repeatedly doing this can produce a high arousal state and even euphoria. Unfortunately it usually ends with a terrible come-down into even more severe depression.

Other means of stimulating arousal level are listed in Table 2. For those of us who find the excessively loud music at discotheques painful on our ears, it is difficult to realize that this is used by some young people as a form of brain stimulation. Small degrees of depression can be masked by this form of arousal-stimulating technique.

The use of challenges to authority as a form of excitement is not widely recognized. Defiance at home only serves to raise arousal level if it leads to some sort of argument or there is the suspense

Table 2. Stimulation of Arousal to Mask Depression

Sleep deprivation

Starvation - anorexia nervosa

Constant work: inventing jobs to do

Rows with spouse

Very loud music (discotheques)

Challenging authority
- home
- school
- law

Violent fights

Self injury - slashing
- acid
- cigarette burns

Drugs - caffeine
- nicotine
- amphetamine

of wondering if one will be found out. At school the rewards are much greater because when a disturbance is produced in the classroom, the other children will often multiply the excitement, especially with certain teachers. At times very little real work may be done for days on end. Unfortunately the initiator of the disturbance eventually feels the heavy hand of retribution and this may increase the depression markedly. At length, no amount of excitement can overcome the depression felt and in a moment of exhaustion of the coping process an overdose of drugs is likely to be taken.

Many of these young people, after treatment with antidepressants for two or three months may return to the same class and the same teachers and work quite normally.

In some circumstances challenging authority at school may be too easy and not sufficiently exciting. Challenging the law may then be much more rewarding in terms of raising arousal level. The suspense, and perhaps the element of the unknown concerning what would happen if caught, certainly is as effective or more so than watching such things on films or television. The studies of Levi and his colleagues (1972) have shown quite clearly thc increase in adrenaline excretion in those watching such "exciting" films: there is no doubt that the real life enactment would produce at least an equal adrenaline response.

The release of adrenaline is not only an indication that the arousal level has been stimulated but it is also a potentiator because it still further excites the reticular formation which leads to further enhancement of behavioral arousal.

The use of self-injury as a form of mental stimulation probably falls into a special category. The suspense until they do the cutting or burning is a phase during which excitement rises but the actual self-damage is essential to trigger off the release of sufficient endorphin ("endogenous morphine") to make them insensitive to pain. Although they feel the cutting or burning they have no pain sensation. Indeed the constant repetition of these acts may well become an addiction so as to get repeated releases of endorphin.

The same probably applies to those who are involved in brutal violence, particularly kicking the person in the face. At the moment of doing so it is as if it is happening to the assailant and so the endorphin is released. In some teenagers it appears that taking part in such violence becomes the equivalent of a shot of heroin. Indeed, the uncertainty of the extent of retaliation may well heighten the excitement and the endorphin response. Our studies of wife-batterers suggest that it takes three to six months' treatment with highly sedative antidepressants to get them out of the high arousal state in which violence is an almost automatic, unconscious act.

Two drugs are in everyday use because of their mental stimulating effects: these are caffeine and nicotine. Within limits caffeine has a useful stimulating effect when great demands upon mental reserves are required. Only occasionally is it taken to the point of tremor and incoordination. Nicotine has frequently been shown to improve performance in vigilance tests and in delaying the onset of fatigue (Schachter, 1977). In our own studies it is surprising that some heavy smokers whose performance in tests is consistently worse after smoking, are unaware that they have reached the point of negative returns. Presumably the nicotine is having some other effect on the brain at this time.

## FEATURES OF FAILURE OF COPING

The common phenomena which are found in people whose coping powers are pushed to near the limit are listed in Table 3. Sleep disturbance and irritability are particularly common features. As they move towards a depressed state, whether overt or masked, efficiency begins to fall. Among the more determined are those who work longer and longer hours with less and less result.

It is in the more determined people, or those on whom challenges fall regardless of the care they may take, that the more marked aspects of coping failure are seen. A change in menstrual pattern may occur and persist in some women, often associated with loss of libido. One of the factors in motivating high arousal may be to get some restoration or even heightening of libido. Impotence in men is mostly a reflection of driving the coping mechanism too far.

More severe changes occur in those who begin to show overt depression, such as crying attacks, verbal or physical abuse and resort to excessive use of a variety of drugs, especially alcohol and tranquilizers.

Table 3. Features of Coping Failure

Sleep disturbance

Irritability

Lack of concentration

Menstrual disturbance

Loss of libido

Impotence

Crying attacks

Unprovoked verbal or physical abuse

Depression

Excessive use of drugs

## TREATMENT OF COPING FAILURE

The drug therapy most commonly used is with tranquilizers. A high proportion of people we see with coping failure have been on tranquilizers for some time with no obvious benefit. However, withdrawal from tranquilizers may produce very unpleasant effects. Antidepressants are much more effective in enhancing coping ability though, as in the treatment of depression, they take some weeks to get to a maximum effect and usually have to be continued for several months.

Of much greater importance is realizing the mechanisms which lead to erosion of coping powers and adapting one's life to avoid, as far as possible, the sort of challenges which will overtax the coping process. Unfortunately this so often means some loss of money as a second job is given up or the mother of a young family has to stop working the "twilight" shift between 6 p.m. and 10 p.m. Eventually some can be persuaded that a calmer, happier life is frequently possible if some of the drive is taken off and the limbic system of the brain is allowed some periods without being in over-drive.

## REFERENCES

Benedict, F. G., 1915, "A Study of Prolonged Fasting", Carnegie Institution of Washington, Washington, D.C.

Brown, G. W. and Harris, T., 1978, "Social Origins of Depression", Tavistock Publications, London.

Levi, L., 1972, "Stress and Distress in Response to Psychosocial Stimuli", Pergamon, Oxford.

Ludbrook, J., Vincent, A., and Walsh, J. A., 1975, Effects of mental arithmetic on arterial pressure and hand blood flow. Clin. Exper. Pharmac. Physiol. Suppl. 2:67.

Pollitt, J., and Young, J., 1971, Anxiety state or masked depression? Brit. Jnl. Psychiat. 119:143.

Schachter, S., 1977, Nicotine regulation in heavy and light smokers, Jnl. Exp. Psych. Gen. 106:5.

## CIVIC EDUCATION IN A STRESSFUL SOCIETY:

## A PROGRAM OF VALUE CLARITY AND TENSION REDUCTION

William G. Williams, Ed.D.

Department of Education
Eastern Wesleyan University
Cheney, Washington

The area of education loosely labeled civic education has as one of its major goals the development of citizens that will preserve and extend democratic values. The schools, however, have tended to ignore the totality of experiences which are essential for the making of good citizens. The compartmentalization of the curriculum has narrowly focused civic education in a formal class called social studies.

There is a growing body of research which links low self-esteem to anti-democratic behavior. In addition there is an increasing amount of research which relates social stress to the lowering of self-esteem. Current technological society provides a wide variety of social stresses which are constant, wearing, and cumulative. The knowledge of the effects of these stresses upon mental and physical health and ultimately upon self-esteem and democratic citizenship has had little impact on school curriculum. There needs to be a psychological and physical dimension to civic education as well as a cognitive one. Civic education needs to focus on ways of developing positive coping abilities which promote physical relaxation and psychological balance. High self-esteem and democratic behavior depend on these abilities.

The literature relating personality traits to political beliefs and behaviors is voluminous (Greenstein and Learner, 1971). Certain scholars, however, have narrowed their focus to those traits necessary for democratic commitment. Harold Lasswell (1951), one of the early pioneers in this endeavor, attempted to identify the democratic character. According to Lasswell, all the democratic character traits came from a common source, the individual's positive estimation of himself. The reason democratic character did not develop was because low estimates of the self were permitted to form.

Inkeles (1961) drew a similar picture of the democratic personality. The democrat was confident of his own self-worth and the values of others; he was flexible, tolerant of ambiguity and differences, open minded, and relatively free from anxiety. These traits caused the individual to be well integrated psychologically and socially.

Lane (1962), although stating his position negatively, outlined the beliefs, needs, patterns of behavior, and psychological states which diminished a person's desire or capacity to be a democrat. Among the many pathologies listed were alienation from society, pervasive cynicism, irrationality, self-estrangement, and loss of identity. All of the pathologies cohered and formed a distinctive psychological type, concluded Lane, the impoverished self. The impoverished self was built from a composite of low self-acceptance, low self-esteem, and low ego strength.

After reviewing the literature relating personality traits to democratic behavior, Sniderman (1975) noticed the emphasis each scholar gave to the relationship between positive self-esteem and democratic behavior. In addition he found a number of research studies which showed low self-esteem a significant cause of conformity (Gergen and Bauer, 1967), psychological maladjustment (Smith, 1958), poor school achievement (Crandall, 1966), and racial discrimination (Heiss and Owens, 1972). Sniderman decided to put the low self-esteem, anti-democratic behavior theory to empirical test.

Identifying personal unworthiness, interpersonal competence and status inferiority as the three components of self-esteem, he analyzed the data drawn from two studies done by Herbert McClosky (1968). After correlating levels of self-esteem with a variety of social and political attitudes, Sniderman agreed with the earlier theoretical conclusion. "The evidence seems plain, the conclusion obvious," he declared:

> Low self-esteem encourages a susceptibility to political extremism. Compared to those with high self-esteem, those with low self-esteem show markedly less tolerance, less support for procedural rights, less faith in democracy, and more cynicism about politics. They have a penchant for seeing conspiracies at work, a disenchantment with the established political order, an express desire for large-scale change by whatever means possible, at whatever cost necessary. They set little store by freedom of speech and assembly (unless it is theirs), the importance of diversity in an open society, the principle of equality.

Sniderman softened his position somewhat, adding that individuals with low self-esteem were less likely to participate in politics and, therefore, less susceptible to extremist views. Yet this was hardly a positive statement as democratic society depends on the active involvement of large numbers of citizens.

If these scholars are correct in their conclusion, if democratic behavior is a by-product of high self-esteem, it follows that civic education should be centrally concerned with its development and maintenance. But just how susceptible is self-esteem to change, and what effect does social stress have upon it? Research does not always answer these questions with consistency.*

The literature regarding personality theory, of which self-esteem is a part, is extensive but contradictory. One of the basic disputes concerns the malleability of personality traits. Individual or consistency theories believe that basic personality is formed at a very young age, and then stability occurs; social theories, however, focus on events outside the individual and emphasize continuous change throughout a person's lifetime (Bavelas, 1978).

Probably the greatest influence on the acceptance of the stability theory as it relates to self-esteem has been the work of Coopersmith (1967). His eight-year longitudinal study was, and is, the definitive study in self-esteem. Coopersmith admitted there were transitory changes in self-esteem, but he thought them momentary, situational, and limited. He based his conclusions on two studies: (1) a study by Aronson and Mills (1959) who admitted that specific incidents and environmental changes did produce shifts in self-esteem, but who concluded that self-esteem reverted to its customary level when conditions returned to normal, and (2) his own study which found that over a three-year period, a group of fifth graders showed consistency in self-esteem levels. Coopersmith concluded that he was in agreement with the consistency theory of personality development.

Yet the consistency theory regarding self-esteem has come under recent criticism. Jones (1973), after reviewing sixteen research studies relating to self-esteem, concluded that only six supported

*One of the difficulties in discussing self-esteem is that it has been examined under so many labels including self-concept, self-esteem, self-image and self-evaluation (Wylie, 1961). Many of the studies cover only one aspect of what is generally thought to be self-esteem. Coopersmith's (1967) definition of self-esteem as "a personal judgment of worthiness that is expressed in the attitudes the individual holds toward himself" seems a helpful working definition and appears to cover what most researchers are trying to get at.

the consistency theory and that the support of these six was questionable. There is also a growing body of research suggesting self-esteem does change with changing environmental conditions (Aronson and Mettee, 1968; Freedman and Doob, 1969; Golin, Hartman, Klatt, Munz and Wolfgang, 1977; Ludwig and Maehr, 1967; McMillan, 1968; McMillan and Helmrich, 1969; McMillan and Renolds, 1969; Wilcox and Mitchell, 1977). It appears, therefore, that the early years are extremely important in the formation of self-esteem and that self-esteem is one of the more stable individual characteristics. Yet it also appears, given the right environmental conditions, self-esteem can be raised or lowered throughout a person's lifetime.

What effect does stress have upon self-esteem?* Disapproval treatment, rejection or negative feedback, which many individuals interpret as being stressful, when used in laboratory research has produced lowered self-esteem. Ludwig and Maehr (1967) found that seventh and eighth-grade boys, when given disapproval treatment for performing various physical tasks, showed lowered self-esteem. Gibby and Gibby (1967) explored the effects of academic failure upon seventh grade students. Under the failure situation, students regarded themselves less highly and believed they were not as highly regarded by others. Wilcox and Mitchell (1977), using a role playing exercise, found that rejected college students showed a decrease in self-esteem.

Stressful field conditions also seem to produce lowered self-esteem. Grinker and Spiegel (1945) found that a basic effect of combat was a loss of self-confidence regarding personal invulnerability. Schmideberg (1942) found similar results among victims of bombing raids, and Wolfenstein (1957) reported the same effect among survivors of natural disasters. Helmreich (1972), basing his conclusions on circumstantial evidence, reviewed a number of studies which examined peer group influence in stress situations. These studies, he concluded, revealed behaviors typical of persons suffering from loss of self-esteem.

---

*Stress as used in this paper is defined as "a stimulus or condition that produces demands on the human organism that require it to exceed its ordinary level of functioning or that restrict activity levels below usual levels of functioning" (Scott and Howard, 1970). Notice that the definition allows for both psychological and physical reactions to conditions, and that it includes nontraumatic, wearing events as well as traumatic ones. Also, a situation of boredom or of sensory deprivation is included. In addition, the definition allows for individual differences since it allows for the activity level at which each person most comfortably functions.

What is the reaction of individual self-esteem to long-term social stress, to the cumulative and wearing events of most modern industrial democracies? Here the answers are not quite so clear. Scott (1967) concluded, after studying the patterns of illness in a group of female employees, that nontraumatic but long-term wearing events produced the same kinds of physiological and psychological responses to stress as traumatic situations. The research of Brown (1974), Dohrenwend and Dohrenwend (1969), and Holms and Rahe (1967) has focused on the physical and psychological effects of specific life events. Their conclusions indicate that cumulative life changes can result in mental and physical illness. Janis (1971), after examining the literature relating to long-term stress, reasoned that the same kind of change produced by a single disaster or traumatic event could also develop gradually if a highly stressful life situation continued for a prolonged period. An individual's basic attitude of self-confidence about coping, he reasoned, could be severely shaken by "an accumulation of . . . stresses over a long period of time."

Two more recent studies shed additional light on the effect of long-term stress on self-esteem. Shanan, De-Nour, and Garty (1976) examined the effects of prolonged stress upon coping style in terminal renal failure patients. The readiness to cope actively with challenging or threatening situations was found dramatically reduced and a shift from positive self-perceptions to negative ones occurred. Chronological age or social background was found unrelated to coping behavior. Shanan and his associates concluded that prolonged stress led to negative self-concepts and passive coping styles.

Frankenhaeuser and Gardell (1976) found similar results of stress upon self-esteem in an interesting study examining the effect of overload and underload work factors on well-being, job satisfaction, and health. They indicated the data presented was representative of work conditions in a wide range of industries. The machine paced work, and the lack of control over the work, they concluded, was a serious threat to self-esteem.

At this point we cannot say with absolute certainty that prolonged social stress, the kind produced by modern technological society, does lower self-esteem, but research and common logic certainly point in that direction. And it does appear that when social conditions are ripe, the effects of lowered self-esteem do spill over into the political and social arena in the form of antidemocratic behavior.

Are the social conditions ripe? If we are to believe the sociologists and the host of other social philosophers examining current technological society, social stress is constant and ubiquitous and responsible for a variety of maladaptive behaviors (Ellul, 1967; Hoffer, 1964; Marcuse, 1964; Schumacher, 1977; Toffler, 1970).

It is not necessary here to examine in detail the modern social stresses to which human beings are exposed, but perhaps it would be helpful to sketch in broad strokes some current conditions relating to social stress, remembering that not all individuals will interpret the same event or condition as stressful. It is possible, however, to refer to those events or conditions most likely to produce disturbances in people.

Disturbances seem at the center of the family unit of today. The family unit has undergone major changes over the past century. The nuclear family of today offers much less insulation from social stress than did the extended family of the Nineteenth Century. Members experience less restraint, but they are exposed to more conflict. There is less cohesion in the family and more ambivalence. Recent estimates suggest that in the United States two out of every five families contains only one parent.

Children particularly experience isolation. They encounter few adults as compared to societies with extended families. Until the child goes to school, the only adults he encounters besides the parents are relatives and mothers of playmates. There is, of course, the vicarious experience with the television, and the child does interact with the teacher when he goes to school, but in general childhood experience does not lead easily and smoothly into adult life. The child experiences few economic or social responsibilities; his play does not prepare him for his occupation, and his formal education is often abstract and divorced from life experiences. Children are expected to obey adult demands, but they are also expected to be self-assertive in order to behave like adults. They are given conflicting information on restraining impulses that adults are freely allowed to express. Technological society has created a mass sub-culture called adolescence with its own values and behaviors.

The adult male also feels the stresses of modern society. The father's position in the family has changed considerably over the past century. In order to provide an acceptable living standard, he must compete with other workers. His work environment often offers few rewards, yet it demands time and effort. When he fails, he looses self-esteem in the work setting as well as in the family. And even when he provides well, he often receives little family affection.

The woman of the Twentieth Century, however, has experienced emancipation, for no longer is she limited to the career of homemaker. Modern technological developments have made homelife easier and less stressful, and the advent of birth control measures has freed the mother to devote more time to her own interests. Yet all is not well. Women, too, are thrust into the competition of the work environment, often suffering the same social stresses as the male. In addition, she if often confused over roles, not exactly sure what being feminine and female means.

The work environment in Twentieth Century society is also one of stress. People congest in large cities working for impersonal companies or governments. They hurry to and from work engaging in work that is often personally unsatisfying and under conditions that could be labeled inhumane. Natural bodily rhythms are subjected to clock time, and the noise of the factory often impedes communications. White collar co-workers are frequently competitors, while labor and management engage in posturing and confrontation.

Finally, modern society is one of rapid change. Social change in general is stressful. Occupation and residence shifts, economic and political upheavals, and high speed technological changes all place increased physical and psychological demands upon people. And modern mass media makes us aware of stressful events outside our local community. We are exposed to a wide variety of world-wide situations that in former times would have gone unnoticed.

The foregoing is a limited subjective analysis of the current social scene drawn in part from the writings of Groen and Bastiaans (1975), Kneller (1965), and Ryan (1969). And some of the conditions described are overdrawn for not all individuals experience these social stresses, and many that do are able to cope and to maintain high levels of self-esteem. Nevertheless, for large numbers of people, the wearing social stresses of modern industrial society do create psychological imbalance and physical tension, ultimately leading to loss of self-esteem and to anti-democratic behavior.

What can civic education do about all this? Certainly the foregoing suggests that one effort should be to aid students in the development of high self-esteem. High self-esteem seems to carry with it some of the insulation necessary to cope successfully with the social stresses of modern society (Coopersmith, 1967). But beyond the development of high self-esteem, education needs to search for techniques for building effective ways of dealing with social stress in order that high self-esteem can be maintained.*

---

*I do not wish to minimize the importance of developing good self-esteem, but the emphasis of this paper is on developing coping abilities in order that high levels of self-esteem can be maintained. Interestingly, in helping children and adolescents learn to cope with stress, a concomitant result is that higher levels of self-esteem are built (Cohen, 1964). However, the building of high self-esteem goes beyond the learning of coping skills. The development of self-esteem is a result of the complex interaction of the individual with parents, peer, and adults.

Coopersmith (1968) has suggested that we need to give more attention to building the capacity "to respond constructively to challenges and troublesome conditions . . ." His suggestion seems sound.

Stress researchers use the term "cope" when referring to an individual's attempt to respond to challenging and troublesome conditions. Coping, however, should not be confused with simply adapting. Teaching children to cope with stress does not teach them to simply accept social conditions and then to live in a negative way. Coping compares favorably with the problem-solving process. It assimilates new information, corrects when necessary, and then accommodates to new situations (Haan, 1977; Janis and Mann, 1977). It does not teach individuals to opt for the status quo, nor does it teach individuals to blindly accept change; it does not support a particular social or economic bias. It does, however, support the democratic faith in that it is consistent with rational, democratic problem solving.

One area where schools need to focus attention if children are to develop positive coping behaviors is in the area of value clarity. Confusion regarding correct decisions is widespread among children, adolescents and adults. People simply do not know what they believe; they have no basis upon which to make judgments. Many of the stress related problems are really value problems. People are buffeted by social stress because they have not developed the inner conviction of what is to be valued (Howe and Howe, 1975; Raths, Harmin and Simon, 1978; Reisman, Denney and Glazer, 1950).

Value clarification, a process developed by Louis Raths and his associates (Raths, Harmin and Simon, 1966), is a technique that seems to hold promise in contributing to coping abilities and to stable high self-esteem. Popularized through the writings and workshops of Sidney Simon, the clarification process has influenced teachers at all levels of education. Raths and Simon posit the belief that the irrationality, apathy, and confusion of Western society is the result of rapid social upheaval. At the root of this maladaptive behavior is the problem of value confusion. Adults and youth alike do not know what they are for or what is worth working for. The function of the teacher, using value clarification techniques, is to constantly question students concerning their goals, aspirations, attitudes, beliefs, and conclusions, to ask them why they have chosen what they have chosen. The process is one where the student is constantly called upon to make choices relating to personal and social events and to defend his choices based on a rational explanation of his value preferences. Simon and others (Howe and Howe, 1975; Simon, Howe, and Kirschenbaum, 1972) have devised numerous activities to use within the classroom to stimulate the clarification process.

Raths et al. (1978) have concluded that many students after experiencing value clarification show less apathy and conformity and more independence and seriousness of purpose. In addition, students display an increase in self-direction and self-trust. Other positive results include a reduction in uncertainty, inconsistency, overdissention and disruptive behavior. And particularly important from the standpoint of positive coping, students show an increased confidence that problems can be solved and personal power can be marshalled. A number of research studies seem to confirm these conclusions (Blokker, Glaser and Kirschenbaum, 1976; Covault, 1973; Gorsuch, Arno and Bachelder, 1976; Guziak, 1974; Kelly 1976; Smith, 1973; Wilgoren, 1973).

Value clarification, it seems, prepares the student for many of the social stresses he will encounter and that will demand coping. Preparedness reduces anxiety and frustration. The student knows what he believes and choices become easier and less stressful (Lazarus, 1977). Also, the student by engaging in value clarification has been involved in the problem solving process. He has learned how to deal rationally and constructively with stressful or problem situations. If handled correctly by the teacher, value clarification exposes the student to a variety of personal and social situations and issues similar to ones he will encounter outside the classroom. Antonovsky (1974) has suggested that the individual's ability to cope is based in part on a concept called homeostatic flexibility, which he defines as the ability to accept alternatives. Value clarification gives the student practice in confronting a wide variety of situations and in selecting from a large number of alternatives. Value clarification leads to the development of homoostatic flexibility.

Another strategy, similar to value clarification, is a technique which causes the student to confront moral dilemmas. Based on the moral development theory of Lawrence Kohlberg (1971), moral dilemma strategy presents a personal or social situation to students which demands a solution based on moral reasoning. There are, of course, a variety of solutions for each dilemma, and there are no right answers. The role of the teacher is to create moral conflict and cognitive disequilibrium among the students. Students are to intellectually reason through their choices and are to engage in discussion with fellow students (Hersh, Paolitto, and Reimer, 1979). Although Kohlberg's developmental theory has undergone some telling philosophical and empirical criticism and no longer appears as valid as it once did (Kurtiness and Greif, 1974) the use of moral dilemmas still appears a useful technique in developing successful coping abilities. Many of the same benefits which result from value clarification also result from confronting moral dilemmas. In addition moral dilemmas offer the students situations filled with ambiguity. Lazarus (1966) has suggested that successful coping in part depends on the individual's ability to resolve the ambiguity of a situation. Moral dilemmas give the students practice in resolving ambiguities.

There are, however, some serious objections to a civic education program using only value clarification (Colby, 1975; Stewart, 1975). And the same objections would apply to moral dilemma techniques when stripped of Kohlberg's theoretical base. It seems obvious that as a way of helping students clarify and cope with what is often a confusing and bewildering variety of choices, clarification techniques and moral dilemma strategies holds great promise. Yet the vagueness concerning what values students tend to internalize creates a social as well as a philosophical problem. Recent behavior at the highest levels of government shows the emptiness of such a relativistic position. When human beings are resolving stressful personal and social issues, we want them to resolve the issues in ways that will further humane and rational goals.

Perhaps a necessary adjunct to value clarification might be what Lawrence Cremin, rephrasing Mathew Arnold, has called the need to "encourage universal acquaintance with the best that has been thought and said" (Cremin, 1965). Cremin in his "Genius of American Education" suggested that the school was uniquely equipped to make students aware of "the constant bombardment of facts, opinions and values to which they are subjected and to help them question what they see and hear . . ." Ultimately, he concluded, schools needed to provide the intellectual resources needed "to make judgments and to assess significance."

Cremin's suggestion fills the void inherent in the value clarification process. Human beings do not internalize values devoid of environmental influence, Cremin's concern is that schools as one influence should opt on the side of the rational and humane values. To so believe goes to the very heart of a major philosophical issue. It is not the purpose here to pursue this axiological argument. Suffice to say that a number of scholars have raised serious questions about crude relativism (Van Tassel, 1967). The 1976 National Conference on Citizenship Education devoted its major effort to exploring the question of public and individual morality; as a result the Salt Lake City, Utah, School District identified twelve democratic principles (values) to be taught as guides to behavior or, to use Cremin's terms, as resources to make judgments and to assess significance (Thomas and Richards, 1979).

Much of this sounds quite traditional. Civic education has often attempted to teach the best that has been thought and said as guides to behavior. Yet often it has been a kind of education using dull and unimaginative techniques, an education attempting to bludgeon into students the best that has been thought and said. We need to make students aware of what is rational and humane, but we also need to soften our pedagogy. Students could be shown that civilized behavior has often been measured by the humane and rational values. They could then be asked to consider these ideals as guides to individual and social behavior. We not only want students to cope with the stresses of the social environment, we want them to cope making choices that will further positive individual and social ends. Value clarification remains silent on what values students should choose. What is needed, it appears, is an artful meshing of Cremin's universal acquaintance with Raths and Simons' value clarification.

Yet clarity of values consistent with humane and rational goals is but a partial answer to meeting the stresses of modern technological society. Being clear about what one believes certainly does contribute to coping abilities and to the maintenance of high self-esteem, but even this cognitive and psychological insulation does not provide the physical resources necessary to deal with social stress. Shalit (1977), has suggested that "the failure to resolve ambiguity, or only partial resolution of ambiguity might well set the upper limit to the success of the whole coping process." Ambiguity, however, is at the very center of democratic society. The democratic faith, by the nature of the principles it affirms, is a constant stimulus to change. It encourages people to speak their minds and to act on their beliefs. By being open, it throws its citizens into conflict. And many of the tenets of the democratic faith are themselves ambiguous. How should a democratic society balance the claims of the majority against the rights of a minority? Are certain rights more basic than others, and which should take precedence in event of conflict? To live in a democratic society is to live with stress (Williams, 1972). Even if one is clear about the values one holds, social stress will still exist. Anyone attempting to work within the democratic system will experience conflict and ambiguity and will be subjected to its psychological and physical demands. Psychological balance and the maintenance of high self-esteem will not be achieved by value clarity alone.

It is widely recognized that reactions to stress are physiological as well as psychological (Dohrenwend and Dohrenwend, 1974; Jacobson, 1964; Monat and Lazarus, 1977). Negative psychological reactions to stress may also trigger negative physiological responses. Anxiety and fear, for example, may be expressed not only through subjective feelings of intense dread and discomfort, but also through altercations in basic physiological processes (Alexander, 1950; Crider, 1970; Groen and Bastiaans, 1975). Conversely, prolonged physical tension can negatively regulate psychological and social performance (Jacobson, 1964). It appears that the physiological, psychological, and social systems are linked. Stress reaction in one system has ramifications in the other (Caudill, 1961).

It follows, therefore, that if the individual is going to cope with stress effectively, he must be taught ways of handling physical tension. Civic education for the maintenance of high self-esteem is not only cognitive and psychological in character, it is also physiological. Ways of controlling physical tension are as important to democratic behavior as are cognitive understandings of the democratic process. Educators working in the area of tension control are civic educators. Our failure in education has been the inability to see the inter-locking relationships of the cognitive, psychological, and physical areas, all of which play a part in the total education of the democratic citizen.

It is not the purpose here to examine in detail the variety of tension control techniques. The literature examining bio-feedback, meditation, progressive relaxation, and physical exercise as successful ways of managing tension is immense and growing. However, several suggestions can be made relating tension control to education in the schools.

Although the use of biofeedback (Schwartz and Beatty, 1977) and meditation techniques (Wallace, 1970) seem to be effective in helping to control tension, their use in the schools seems limited. Biofeedback uses sophisticated electronic instruments to teach individuals to control their internal processes, but the cost of these instruments seems prohibitive for most school systems. Meditation, in many minds, is associated with various religious and mystical cults. Parents are not yet ready to accept at the elementary or secondary level the teaching of meditation techniques even though as Herbert Benson (1975) has shown, meditation need not be mystical or religious.

The most promising area for teaching tension control in the schools seems to lie in the area of progressive relaxation. Pioneered by Edmund Jacobson (1929) and made popular to physical educators through the efforts of Arthur Steinhaus (1963), progressive relaxation requires little in the way of mechanical apparatus; nor is it in any way attached to something mystical. It can be taught quite easily in the physical education setting. There are already a number of physical educators in the United States who have been trained in progressive relaxation techniques (Frederick, 1975), and some novel ways of teaching progressive relaxation to children are beginning to appear (Koeppen, 1974).

Very simply, progressive relaxation teaches the individual to recognize both muscle tenseness and muscle relaxation. The individual is taught to achieve relaxation over the external muscles. When this is achieved, internal muscle tension subsides, nerves become inactive, pulse rate declines, temperature and blood pressure fall and mental and emotional activity diminish. This deep state of relaxation produces a quiescence of the entire body. The individual goes beyond the normal degree of relaxation which usually contains some residual tension. Progressive relaxation requires practice, and it is not simply learned in a matter of days. The process can lead to a state where total relaxation of the body is achieved. It can also produce the ability to relax muscles not required when the individual is engaged in every day tasks. This latter ability, called differential relaxation, seems most beneficial in helping the individual cope with stress. He is taught to minimize tension when dealing with stressful situations; the individual's ability to cope seems enhanced (Jacobson, 1929, 1964, 1970). There are numerous reports of personal cases where progressive relaxation proved highly successful (Jacobson, 1970). Progressive relaxation, it appears, should be a necessary and integral part of a total civic education program.

Another area receiving increasing attention for achieving physical and mental relaxation is the use of physical exercise. Conventional wisdom, for many years, has suggested that exercise produced a calming effect upon the body, but there has been little empirical research to support this conclusion. Recently some research has begun to demonstrate the beneficial relaxation results of physical exercise (deVries, 1975). At this point, the results are tentative, and one wishes the exercise physiologists would provide us with more information. If one is to believe the thousands of personal testimonials found in such popular books as James Fixx's "The Complete Book of Running" or in the popular periodicals such as Runner's World, certainly something positive is happening.

A few studies have been done relating mental health and physical exercise. Michael (1957) found that a physical fitness program increased ability to withstand emotional stress, while Jette (1971) determined that habitual exercisers were less anxious than nonexercisers. In a series of studies, Ismail and Young (1973, 1974, 1976, 1977) repeatedly found a positive relationship between physical fitness and such personality characteristics as emotional stability, self-confidence, and security. Herbert deVries has focused his attention on the direct relationship between exercise and neuromuscular tension (1968, 1970, 1972). In all results, he found moderate exercise reduced tension. His research study in 1972 used individuals with anxiety-tension problems. Exercise of the appropriate type and at the correct level of intensity, he found, had a significantly greater effect upon reduced tension than did a frequently prescribed tranquilizing drug. DeVries cautiously concluded, after examining the research relating physical exercise to relaxation, that rhythmic exercise such as jogging, cycling, or bench stepping with a duration of from five to ten minutes at thirty to fifty percent of maximum was most effective in producing the tranquilizing effect (1975).

One cannot state with certainty that exercise in general reduces muscular tension and leads to physical and mental relaxation, but the literature is certainly suggestive. What might prove ultimately beneficial is a program combining the teaching of progressive relaxation techniques along with the development of life-long exercise habits. Again such a program would contribute significantly to the over-all goal of democratic civic education.

It seems clear that we need to see civic education beyond the bounds of the traditional cognitive approach. Civic education should not be compartmentalized into a social studies class. Civic education for a democratic society needs to link the social, psychological and physical lives of people. The foregoing has argued that anti-democratic behavior is often a result of low self-esteem. It has been further shown that prolonged wearing social stress can lead to low self-esteem. A program focusing on value clarity and upon tension reduction has been suggested as ways to further coping abilities and to help maintain good self-esteem.

Modern technological society has produced a variety of social stresses, but even if these irritants were eliminated, stress would still be with us; democratic society is inherently stressful. Yet for all its messy ambiguities, democratic society is the one in which most of us would choose to live. Its stresses for some are invigorating and motivating; these individuals have learned how to cope effectively. Many, however, are not so successful. The preservation and extension of democratic society might well rest on the ability of civic educators to help all individuals cope with social stress in a positive and productive way.

## REFERENCES

Alexander, F., 1950, "Psychosomatic Medicine, Its Principles and Applications," Norton, New York.

Antonovsky, A., 1974, Conceptual and methodological problems in stressful life events: the study of resistance to stressful life events, in "Stressful Life Events: Their Nature and Effects," B. S. Dohrenwend and B. P. Dohrenwend, eds., John Wiley and Sons, New York.

Aronson, E., and Mettee, D., 1968, Dishonest behavior as a function of differential levels of induced self-esteem, Jnl. of Pers. and Soc. Psych., 9:121.

Aronson, E., and Mills, J., 1959, The effects of severity of initiation on liking for a group, Jnl. of Abn. Soc. Psych., 59:177.

Bavelas, J. B., 1978, "Personality: Current Theory and Research," Brooks/Cole Publishing Co., Monterey, Calif.

Benson, H., 1975, "The Relaxation Response," William Morrow, New York.

Blokker, Glaser, and Kirschenbaum, H., 1976, Unpublished manuscript.

Brown, G. W., 1974, Meaning, measurement and stress of life events, in "Stressful Life Events: Their Nature and Effects," B. S. Dohrenwend and B. P. Dohrenwend, eds., John Wiley and Sons, New York.

Caudill, W., 1961, Effects of social and cultural systems in reacting to stress, N.Y. Soc. Sci. Res. Counc., 26:51.

Cohen, A. R., 1964, "Attitude Change and Social Influence," Basic Books, New York.

Colby, A., 1975, Review of "Values and Teaching", in Harvard Ed. Rev., 45:134.

Coopersmith, S., 1968, Studies in self-esteem, Sci. Am., 218:96.

Coopersmith, S., 1967, "The Antecedents of Self-Esteem," W. H. Freeman and Co., San Francisco.

Covault, T., 1973, The application of value clarification teaching strategies with fifth-grade students to investigate their influence on students' self-concept and related classroom coping and interacting behaviors, Unpublished doctoral dissertation, Ohio State University, Columbus.

Crandall, V. C., 1966, Personality characteristics and social and achievement behaviors associated with children's social desirability response tendencies, Jnl. of Pers. and Soc. Psych., 4:477.

Cremin, L. A., 1965, "The Genius of American Education," Random House, Inc., New York.

Crider, A., 1973, Experimental studies of conflict-produced stress, in "Social Stress," S. Levine and N. A. Scotch, eds., Aldine Publishing Co., Chicago.

deVries, H. A., and Adams, G. M., 1972, Electromyographic comparison of single doses of exercise and meprobamate as to effect on muscular relaxation, Am. Jnl. of Phys. Med., 51:130.

deVries, H. A., 1968, Immediate and long-term effects of exercise upon resting muscle acting potential level, Jnl. of Sports Med., 8:1.

deVries, H. A., 1975, Physical education, adult fitness programs; does physical activity promote relaxation? Jnl. of Phys. Ed. and Rec., 46:53.

deVries, H. A., 1970, Physiological effects of an exercise training regimine upon men aged 52-88, Jnl. of Geron., 25:325.

Dohrenwend, B. P., and Dohrenwend, B. S., 1969, "Social Status and Psychological Disorder," John Wiley and Sons, New York.

Dohrenwend, B. S., and Dohrenwend, B. P., eds., "Stressful Life Events: Their Nature and Effect," John Wiley and Sons, New York (1974).

Ellul, J., 1964, "The Technological Society," A. Knopf, New York.

Fixx, J. F., 1977, "The Complete Book of Running," Random House, New York.

Frankenhaeuser, M., and Gardell, B., 1976, Underload and overload in working life: outline of a multidisciplinary approach, Jnl. of Hum. Stress, 2:35.

Frederick, A. B., 1975, Biofeedback and tension control, Jnl. of Phys. Ed. and Rec., 46:75.

Freedman, J., and Doob, A. N., 1969, "Deviancy," Academic Press, New York.

Gergen, K. J., and Bauer, R. A., 1967, Interactive effects of self-esteem and task difficulty on social conformity, Jnl. of Pers. and Soc. Psych., 6:16.

Gibby, R. G., Sr., and Gibby, R. G., Jr., 1967, The effects of stress resulting from academic failure, Jnl. of Clin. Psych., 23:35.

Golin, S., Hartman, S. A., Klatt, E. N., Munz, K., and Wolfgang, G. L., 1977, Effects of self-esteem manipulation on arousal and reactions to sad models in depressed and nondepressed college students, Jnl. of Abn. Psych., 86:435.

Gorsuch, R. L., Arno, D., and Bachelder, R. L., 1976, Summary of research and evaluation of the youth values project, 1973-1976, Unpublished manuscript, YMCA, Akron, Ohio.

Greenstein, F. K., and Lerner, M., eds., "A Source Book for the Study of Personality and Politics," Markham Publishing Co., Chicago (1971).

Grinker, R. R., and Spiegel, J. P., 1945, "Men Under Stress," McGraw-Hill, New York.

Groen, J. J., and Bastiaans, J., 1975, Psychosocial stress, inter-human communication and psychomatic disease, in "Stress and Anxiety," Vol. 1, C. D. Speilberger and I. G. Sarason, eds., John Wiley and Sons, New York.

Guziak, S. J., 1974, The use of values clarification strategies with fifth grade students to investigate influence on self-concept and values, Unpublished doctoral dissertation, Ohio State University, Columbus.

Haan, N., 1977, "Coping and Defending: Processes of Self-Environment Organization," Academic Press, New York.

Heiss, J., and Owens, S., 1972, Self-evaluations in blacks and whites, Am. Jnl. of Soc., 78:360.

Helmreich, R., 1972, Stress, self-esteem and attitudes, in "Attitudes, Conflict, and Social Change," B. T. King and E. McGinnies, eds., Academic Press, New York.

Hersh, R. H., Paolitto, D. P, and Reimer, J., 1979, "Promoting Moral Growth from Piaget to Kohlberg," Longman, New York.

Hoffer, E., 1964, "The Ordeal of Change," Harper and Row, New York.

Holmes, T. H., and Rahe, R. H., 1967, The social readjustment rating scale, Jnl. of Psycho. Res., 11:213.

Howe, L. W., and Howe, M. M., 1975, "Personalizing Education: Values Clarification and Beyond," Hart Publishing Co., Inc., New York.

Inkeles, A., 1961, National character and modern political systems, in "Psychological Anthropology: Approaches to Culture and Personality," F. L. K. Hsu, ed., Dorsey Press, Homewood, Ill.

Ismail, A. H., and Young, R. J., 1976, Influence of physical fitness on second and third order personality factors using orthagonal and oblique rotations, Jnl. of Clin. Psych., 32:268.

Ismail, A. H., 1973, The effect of chronic exercise on the personality of middle-aged men by univariate and multivariate approaches, Jnl. of Hum. Ergo., 2:45.

Jacobson, E., 1964, "Anxiety and Tension Control," J. B. Lippincott Co., Philadelphia.

Jacobson, E., 1970, "Modern Treatment of Tense Patients," Charles C. Thomas, Publishers, Springfield, Ill.

Jacobson, E., 1929, "Progressive Relaxation," University of Chicago Press, Chicago.

Janis, I. L., and Mann, L., 1977, "Decision Making: A Psychological Analysis of Conflict, Choice and Commitment," Macmillan, New York.

Janis, I. L. and Mann, L., 1971, "Stress and Frustration," Harcourt, Brace, Jovanovich, Inc., New York.

Jette, M. A., 1971, A blood serum and personality trait profile of habitual exercisers, "Proceedings of the Joint Meeting of the Canadian Association of Sports Science and the American College of Sports Medicine," Canadian Association of Sports Science, Toronto.

Jones, S. C., 1973, Self and interpersonal evaluations: self-esteem theories versus consistency theories, Psych. Bul., 79:185.

Kelly, F. W., 1976, Selected values clarification strategies and elementary school pupils' self-concept, school sentiment and reading achievement, Unpublished doctoral dissertation, Fordham University, New York.

Kneller, G., 1965, "Educational Anthropology: An Introduction," John Wiley and Sons, Inc., New York.

Koeppen, A. S., 1974, Relaxation training for children, Elem. Sch. Guid. and Couns., 9:14.

Kohlberg, L., 1971, Stages of moral development as a basis for moral education, in "Moral Education," C. M. Beck, B. S. Crittenden, and E. V. Sullivan, eds., Newman Press, New York.

Kurtines, W., and Greif, E. B., 1974, The development of moral thought: review and evaluation of Kohlberg's approach, Psych. Bul., 81:453.

Lane, R., 1962, "Political Ideology," The Free Press, New York.

Lasswell, H. D., 1951, "The Political Writings of Harold D. Lasswell," The Free Press, Glencoe, Ill.

Lazarus, R. S., 1977, Cognitive and coping processes in emotion, in "Stress and Coping: An Anthology," A. Monat and R. Lazarus, eds., Columbia University Press, New York.

Lazarus, R. S., 1966, "Psychological Stress and the Coping Process," McGraw-Hill, New York.

Ludwig, D. L., and Maehr, M. L., 1967, Changes in self-concept and stated behavioral preferences, Child Dev., 38:453.

Marcuse, H., 1964, "One-Dimensional Man," Beacon Press, Boston.

McClosky, H., 1968, Political participation and apathy, in "International Encyclopedia of the Social Sciences, D. Sills, ed., Macmillan, New York.

McMillen, D., and Reynolds, J. E., 1969, Self-esteem and the effectiveness of reconciliation techniques following an argument, Psychon. Sci., 17:208.

McMillen, D., and Helmreich, R., 1968, The effectivensss of several types of ingratiation techniques following an argument, Psychon. Sci., 15:207.

McMillen, D., 1968, Application of the gain-loss model of interpersonal attraction to responses to ingratiating behavior following an argument, Unpublished doctoral dissertation, the University of Texas at Austin.

Michael, D., Jr., 1957, Stress adaption through exercise, Res. Quar., 28:50.

Monat, A., and Lazarus, R. S., eds., "Stress and Coping: An Anthology," Columbia University Press, New York (1977).

Raths, L. E., Harmon, M., and Simon, S. B., 1966, "Values and Teaching," Charles E. Merrill Publishing Co., Columbus, Ohio.

Raths, L. E., Harmon, M., and Simon, S. B., 1978, "Values and Teaching" (2nd ed.), Charles E. Merrill Publishing Co., Columbus, Ohio.

Reisman, D., Denney, R., and Glazer, N., 1950, "The Lonely Crowd: A Study of the Changing American Character," Yale University Press, New Haven.

Runners World, 1975-1979, Vols. 10-14.

Ryan, B. F., 1969, "Social and Cultural Change," The Ronald Press Co., New York.

Schmideberg, M., 1942, Some observations on individual reactions to air raids, Internat'l. Jnl. of Psycho., 23:146.

Schumacher, E. F., 1977, "A Guide for the Perplexed," Harper and Row, New York.

Schwartz, G. E., and Beatty, J., "Biofeedback: Theory and Research," Academic Press, New York.

Scott, R. A., 1963, Illness and social role difficulties, Unpublished manuscript.

Scott, R. A., and Howard, A., 1970, Models of stress, in "Social Stress," S. Levine and N. A. Scotch, eds., Aldine Publishing Co., Chicago.

Shalit, B., 1977, Structural ambiguity and limits to coping, Jnl. of Hum. Stress, 3:32.

Shanan, J., De Nour, A. K., and Garty, I., 1976, Effects of prolonged stress on coping style in terminal renal failure patients, Jnl. of Hum. Stress, 2:19.

Simon, S. B., Howe, L. W., and Kirschenbaum, H., 1972, "Values Clarification: A Handbook of Practical Strategies," Hart Publishing Co., New York.

Smith, B. C., 1973, Values clarification in drug education: a comparative study, Jnl. of Drug Edu., 3:369.

Smith, B. M., 1958, Six measures of self-concept discrepancy and instability: their interrelations, reliability, and relations to other personality variables, Jnl. of Consult. Psych., 22:101.

Sniderman, P. M., 1975, "Personality and Democratic Politics," The University of California Press, Berkeley.

Steinhaus, A. H., 1963, "Toward an Understanding of Health and Physical Education," W. C. Brown Co., Publishers, Dubuque, Iowa.

Stewart, J. S., 1975, Clarifying values clarification: a critique, Phi Delta Kappan, 56:684.

Thomas, D., and Richards, M., 1979, Ethics education is possible, Phi Delta Kappan, 60:579.

Toffler, A., 1970, "Future Shock," Random House, New York.

VanTassel, D., ed., "American Thought in the Twentieth Century," Thomas Y. Crowell Co., New York (1967).

Wallace, R. K., 1970, "The Physiological Effects of Transcendental Meditation," MIVPRESS, Los Angeles.

Wilcox, J., and Mitchell, J., 1977, Effects of group acceptance/ rejection of self-esteem levels of individual group members in a task-oriented problem-solving group interaction, Small Group Behav., 8:169.

Wilgoren, R. A., 1973, The relationship between the self-concept of pre-service teachers and two methods of teaching value clarification, Unpublished doctoral dissertation, University of Massachusetts, Amherst.

Williams, W. G., 1972, Democracy: the forgotten innovation, The Clearing House, 47:3.

Wolfenstein, M., 1957, "Disaster," Free Press, New York.

Wylie, R., 1961, "The Self-Concept," University of Nebraska Press, Lincoln.

Young, R. J., and Ismail, A. H., 1977, Comparison of selected physiological and personality variables in regular and nonregular adult male exercises, Res. Quar., 48:617.

# A BRIEF ANALYSIS OF POPULARIZATION OF PROGRESSIVE RELAXATION IN JAPAN

Dr. Toshio Watanabe

Yokohama National University
Yokohama, Japan

ABSTRACT*

Muscular relaxation was first introduced to Japan by Dr. Edmund Jacobson and Dr. A. H. Steinhaus about ten years ago, but its importance was not fully appreciated at that time.

For the first few years, because of the rapid progress of industrialization and the changes which occurred accordingly, the nation has been confronted with the problem of stress.

Meanwhile people have started recognizing the significance of muscular relaxation, and it is now one of the most popular topics in journalism. Unfortunately, there are still only few that can actually practice the method.

There remains an urgent need for it to be more widely spread for the sake of the future.

*Only abstract available.

# STRESS AND CARDIOVASCULAR DISORDERS

# EMOTIONAL STRESS TESTING AND RELAXATION IN CARDIAC REHABILITATION

Wesley E. Sime, M.P.H., Ph.D.

Director, Stress Physiology Laboratory
University of Nebraska
Lincoln, Nebraska

There is considerable interest currently in the relationship between emotional stress and coronary heart disease. Since the beginning of recorded medical history clinicians have suspected that stress may be a precipitating factor in the atherosclerotic disease process. Many of these beliefs were based upon anecdotal evidence citing cases of angina pectoris (Lown, 1977) and voodoo death (Engle, 1971) resulting from severe emotional strain. While this evidence was quite enticing it was not sufficient to establish a casual relationship between emotional stress and atherosclerosis.

Fortunately medical science is very conservative and this early suggestive evidence has not swayed the bulk of traditional therapy toward any extreme or exotic treatment procedures. On the contrary, medicine has failed to recognize some meaningful developments in this area because they either lacked hard physiological data to support the theoretical concepts or they did not appear relevant to coronary risk. More recently the developments in psychology, physiology and psychophysiology have produced "relevancy" for the issues in heart disease risk via the progressive, interdisciplinary efforts in behavioral medicine.

Selye's (1946) early work with animals demonstrating the general adaptation syndrome made the term "stress" very popular. Even before that time Cannon (1935) had conceived similar principles with his description of the "fight or flight" response. More recently, Mason (1968) has shown that the mechanisms and characteristics of a "stress/strain" response are not nearly as simple as Selye had viewed it. He demonstrated that intense psychosocial stimuli could result in two completely different neuroendocrine responses depending upon how the victim perceives the situation. In animal responses the effects of shock avoidance (acutely) psychosocial frustration (chronically) have been clearly related to myocardial damage and infarction.

Unfortunately, similar research in humans is impossible for obvious moral and ethical reasons. Yet there persists an overwhelming need to conduct very careful objective research in a controlled environment. In the past few years several efforts have been put forth in this regard. Lown and Verrier (1976) have demonstrated that the frequency of premature ventricular contractions is influenced by psychologically stressful events in the laboratory. In the "real-life" setting, Taggart et al., (1973) showed that ectopic beats, catecholamine level and triglyceride levels were elevated in recovered "cardiac" patients when speaking before an audience.

Further attempts at standardizing psychological input and monitoring patients in the laboratory were initiated by Schiffer, et al., (1976). They monitored heart rate, ECG and blood pressure while patients took a standardized ego-threatening quiz. Angina patients, hypertensive patients and the executive sub-groups all showed significantly higher heart rate and blood pressure responses than did the asymptomatic patients and the non-executives. The results were intriguing because of the group differences, however, there was not enough solid evidence to suggest tht hyper-reactivity of heart rate and blood pressure was implicated in the pathogenesis of the disease.

The coronary-prone behavior pattern concept represents another attempt at providing an objective assessment of the link between stress and coronary heart disease (CHD). In the past two decades much evidence has been accumulated to support the theory that Type A, aggressive, overly-competitive, hyper-alert, time-conscious, hostile individuals are 2 to 6 times more likely to show evidence of coronary heart disease prematurely than are their Type B, easy-going, relaxed but functionally efficient counterparts.

Some efforts to examine the physiological concommitants of Type A versus Type B individuals have yielded very encouraging results. Dembrowski, et al., (In Press) has shown that Type A male college students exhibited four times higher increase in heart rate and twice the increase in systolic blood pressure response to laboratory challenges than did the Type B students. The results were much less dramatic for female students presumably because the lab challenges appeared less salient to females. On the other hand, one could conclude that the reduced reactivity for young females may be a key to their very low incidence of heart disease relative to males. In addition, it was interesting to note that hostility and verbal competitiveness, two components of the Type A complex, correlated most strongly with the changes in blood pressure and heart rate. Apparently there are some components of the Type A complex which are less well tolerated by the cardiovascular system. When identified more clearly and completely these will require much therapeutic attention in the future.

## PSYCHOPHYSIOLOGICAL (EMOTIONAL) STRESS TESTING

### Subject Preparation

It is important to emphasize the need for a resting baseline condition prior to onset of testing. Mere existence, breathing and functioning, requires some degree of physiological arousal. When these are minimal, as in the normal relaxed individual shortly after awakening, one is considered to be at basal metabolic rate (BMR). The experimenter can never be certain when that state is reached, but it should be held as the desired point from which to begin testing. Deference in this issue assures the experimenter that an unknown element contaminates the procedure even before testing begins.

In order to achieve a BMR condition in all test subjects it is perhaps obvious that relaxation procedures are in order. The first step is to allow the subject time and opportunity for habituation and familiarization with the laboratory setting. This usually requires having test subjects visit the lab at least once before testing to sensitize them to the equipment, personnel and procedures. At the start of the actual test the subject should be assured beyond a doubt that all procedures are innocuous and that the subject may even achieve a state of relaxation heretofore not experienced.

Once the electrodes are attached and the equipment is operational, a rest period of at least ten minutes is invoked. During this period of time the experimenter should use external means to facilitate a "relaxation response" experience. Subjects can be encouraged to fall asleep. Soft music and suggestive phrases can be utilized to minimize the cognitive domain. Physical manipulation of musculature is also possible with the use of a recliner chair equipped with vibrator and roller-massage elements. The minimum provision for support is a simple recliner chair. Head, neck, arms, and legs must be supported in a position which is optimally comfortable for the subjects. In some cases this may require cushioning with pillows or elevating the legs to relieve back strain. The room temperature must be comfortable to the subject, presumably set at 72 to 76 degrees Farenheit.

### Physiological and Biochemical Parameters

A wide range of cardiovascular, autonomic and skeletal-muscle measures have been used in psychophysiological testing. The traditional cardiovascular measures include heart rate, blood pressure and electrocardiogram. Without describing the measures available through catheterization, it has become possible in recent years to obtain similar measures indirectly through non-invasive techniques. Thus via impedance cardiography and echocardiography it is possible to monitor cardiac output, stroke volume, systolic time intervals and myocardial contractility. Estimates of peripheral resistance can be obtained by calculations on cardiac output and blood pressure. Autonomic nervous system activity can also be assessed by monitoring skin resistance or skin conductance. The rate of palmar sweating is a very good indicator of sympathetic outflow and can be measured very accurately. In addition, electromyography of the skeletal musculature provides a very accurate estimate of muscle activity and thus overall oxygen consumption. Biochemical measures include urine and blood catecholamines, serum lipids and free fatty acids.

## Emotional Stress Test Stimuli

Since psychophysiological stress testing is a relatively new procedure in cardiovascular medicine, it seems appropriate to utilize a variety of cognitive tasks. It would be desirable to simulate "real-life" experiences with all degrees of emotional involvement. However, there is no way to create "real-life" experiences and still standardize the input for a heterogeneous population. Therefore, the experimenter is forced to utilize a broad variety of cognitive tasks, at least one of which will presumably touch each subject with some semblance of reality.

Some of the cognitive tasks which have been used in the past include: mental arithmetic, choice reaction time task, viewing a horrible film, listening to a vicious argument on tape, word/color conflict task, competitive tasks, insolvable puzzles, interview focused upon previous emotionally-laden events, and high challenge instructions for a physical task such as cold pressor test or isometric hand grip.

Regardless of what task is utilized the impact on the subject will be determined by the degree of challenge imposed by the experimenter and the level of difficulty imposed by the task. Thus it is important at the outset to utilize maximum challenge and expectancy for excellent performance of the task. Secondarily, but perhaps even more important, is the staging of the task. Previous experience with a similar kind of stress testing, exercise tolerance testing, suggests that the test should be graded from a very low intensity progressively upwards to a level beyond which most subjects can perform. In both exercise testing and emotional testing the subject must continue the task in order to obtain valid responses. Verbal prodding from the experiementer is extremely important for the emotional test to ensure active involvement throughout.

## Preliminary Test Results

Previous results in numerous psychophysiology experiments have demonstrated clearly that physiological arousal is a universal response to cognitively-demanding, frustration-type, competitve tasks (Obrist, et al., 1974; Williams, et al., 1975). It is assumed that these circumstances are generalized to the "real-world", that is, they characterize individuals accurately regardless of whether the task is salient or not. One important factor is how the individual respons uniquely to a progressively more demanding task which involves both low challenge and high challenge circumstances (Dembrowski, et al., In Press). Another factor of great interest is the rapidity with which the individual shows recovery from a given level of physiological response. For example, it is likely that individuals who exhibit slow recovery in blood pressure response to a nonfunctional, low intensity, static, exertional task are at high risk of developing essential hypertension (Jacobson, 1978).

Psychophysiological stress testing is currently being tested as a diagnostic tool in coronary heart disease patients. Heart rate, blood pressure and electrocardiogram were monitored before, during and after an ego-threatening quiz in a group of patients with heart disease (Schiffer, et al., 1976). They found a significant relationship between lability of these parameters and severity of disease.

More recently, this author completed preliminary investigations on a similar population matched with a control group for comparative purposes (Sime, et al., 1977). Group differences between patients and controls were not remarkable in light of Schiffer's findings. However, when the population was subdivided further according to behavior type A/B and habitual exercise patterns, the differences in physiological reactivity became apparent. Patients and controls with type A characteristics and/or low exercise habits showed significantly greater lability than did the type B and/or high exercise participants. Dembrowski, et al., (In Press) found even more preponderant differences in cardiovascular responses between Type A and Type B subjects who were being interviewed and were verbalizing answers to a history quiz. Thus it would appear that these techniques show promise of becoming viable diagnostic tools for detection of coronary-proneness or for risk of recurrent infarction.

## RELAXATION TRAINING IN CARDIAC REHABILITATION

Considering the previous discussion relating physiological reactivity (to stress) and coronary heart disease, it is perhaps logical to assume that therapeutic benefits might be derived from any treatment which reduces physiological reactivity. Aside from pharmaceutical therapy which yields numerous side effects, there are many techniques purportedly effective in reducing physiological responses. Among these are biofeedback, autogenic training, meditation and progressive relaxation. The comparative effectiveness of each is an area of great controversy at present. Many therapists feel that progressive relaxation is one of the foremost in terms of long-term effectiveness. Its only limitation is that it requires extensive training on individuals who must have strong motivation to continue.

Patients recovering from myocardial infarction are excellent candidates for long-term behavioral therapy, such as progressive relaxation. They are frightened by a close encounter with death and strongly motivated to pursue any therapy which holds some promise of extending their lives. Thus it seems highly appropriate to initiate relaxation training into the comprehensive cardiac rehabilitation program as soon as possible after release from the hospital. Many clinicians even find it useful to minimize pain and further myocardial damage in the coronary care unit. Obviously at this stage it is relatively difficult to invoke training techniques which produce immediate therapeutic results.

Comprehensive cardiac rehabilitation programs currently include diet management, smoking cessation, medication and supervised exercise therapy at carefully prescribed levels. The exercise therapy generally requires participation three to five times per week with supervision for about six months. This frequency and period of time would also be sufficient to accomplish fairly effective training in progressive relaxation. Thus it would seem to be appropriate to include relaxation training during each session the patient attended for exercise training.

Previous investigations have suggested that exercise, in and of itself, produces some acute reduction in muscle tension (Sime, 1977). Thus it is logical to assume that exercise might be a "facilitating" factor in the relaxation training process. It is generally understood that patients develop awareness of tension levels easier when overall somatic tension is lower at the outset (Sime, 1978).

Recently this author had a rare opportunity to collaborate with a clinical team to develop a comprehensive cardiac rehabilitation program at a community hospital. With all of the preceeding discussion in mind, we were able to incorporate a relaxation training program at the end of each exercise session. Training was conducted by respiration therapists who were personally supervised by this author. Sensory awareness relaxation training (Sime, 1979), was utilized at the outset followed immediately by group progressive relaxation training. The patients were lying in a supine position on soft gymnasium mats with a 15 inch cushion under the lower legs to relieve strain upon the lower back. Training sessions were 20 minutes in duration, three times a week for a period of six months.

Initially, many of the patients thought the program was ridiculous, but within 1 to 5 sessions the majority had experienced a very pleasant relaxation response. As a result the relaxation session became the highlight of the program and it appears to be a permanent aspect of the total program. Anecdotal cases showed some remarkable results. At least one patient showed decrease in systolic blood pressure of 40 mmHg pre-to-post session. Many other patients reported dramatic effects upon their occupational and domestic situations.

In summary, it appears that psychophysiological stress testing is a viable diagnostic tool which can be considered as an adjunct procedure in detecting some individuals who are coronary-prone or at risk of recurrent infarction. Procedures for psychophysiological testing must include extensive cardiovascular monitoring and standardized high-challenge cognitive tasks. Pursuant to these tests it is very appropriate to utilize relaxation training as a major aspect of the comprehensive cardiac rehabilitation program. Benefits include positive cardiovascular changes and self-reported improvements in personal efficiency.

## REFERENCES


Cannon, W. B., 1935, Stresses and strains of homeostasis, Am. Jnl. of the Med. Sci., 189:1.

Dembrowski, T. M., MacDougall, J. M., Herd, J. A., and Shields, J. L., (in press), Effects of level of challenge on pressor and heart rate response in type A and B subjects, Jnl. of App. Soc. Psy.

Engle, G. L., 1971, Sudden and rapid death during psychologic stress, Annals of Int. Med., 74:771.

Jacobson, E., 1978, "Report on test for hypertensives," Unpublished manuscript.

Lown, B. L., and Verrier, R. L., 1976, Neural activity and ventricular fibrillation, New Eng. Jnl. of Med., 294:1165.

Lown, B., 1977, Verbal conditioning of angina pectoris during exercise testing, Am. Jnl. of Card., 40:630.

Mason, J. W., 1968, A review of psychoendocrine research on the pituitary adrenal cortical system, Psychosomatic Med., 30:576.

Obrist, P. A., Lawler, J. E., Howard, J. L., Smithson, K. W., Martin, P. L., and Manning, J., 1974, Sympathetic influences on cardiac rate and contractility during acute stress in humans, Psychophys., 11:405.

Schiffer, F., Hartley, L. H., Schulman, C. L., and Abelman, W. H., 1976, The quiz electrocardiogram: a new diagnostic and research technique for evaluating the relation between emotional stress and ischemic heart disease, Am. Jnl. of Card., 37:41.

Selye, H., 1946, The general adaptation syndrome and the diseases of adaptation, Jnl. of Clin. Endo., 6:117.

Sime, W. E., Pierrynowsky, M. and Sharratt, M., September, 1977, Relationship of exercise and behavior type (A/B) to physiological response to emotional stress, Paper presented at the Canadian Association of Sport Sciences, Winnipeg, Manitoba.

Sime, W. E., 1977, Acute relief of emotional stress, in "Proceedings of the American Association for the Advancement of Tension Control," F. J. McGuigan, ed., A. A. A. T. C., Louisville, Kentucky.

Sime, W. E., 1977, Sensory awareness relaxation training, in "Proceedings of the American Association for the Advancement of Tension Control," F. J. McGuigan, ed., A. A. A. T. C., Louisville, Kentucky.

Taggert, P., Carruthers, M., and Somerville, W., August 18, 1973, Electrocardiogram, plasma catecholamines and lipids and their modification by oxprenolol when speaking before an audience, Lancet, 341.

Williams, R. B., 1975, Cardiovascular and neurophysiologic correlates of sensory intake and rejection. I. Effect of cognitive tasks, Psychophys., 12:427.

# PHYSICAL ACTIVITY, MOOD AND ANXIETY IN NORMAL AND POST-CORONARY MALES

D. A. Hill, B.Sc., M.C.S.P.

Reader Health Sciences
Ulster Polytechnic Institute
Belfast, Northern Ireland

## INTRODUCTION

The relationships between physical activity and physiological health have been examined extensively. Studies have included observation on physical activity at work (Morris and Crawford, 1958) and prescribed physical activity programs (Hellerstein, 1974). The effects of such activity on affective states has not received such widespread attention, perhaps because the variables concerned are more difficult to identify and measure. Some attempts have however been made in this direction (Ismail and Trachman,1973).

This paper consists of two parts. The first part deals with a group of subjects who attended regular exercise twice weekly for nine months. The second part deals with a group of patients who recently suffered myocardial infarction.

## PART 1

In the late summer of 1971 a group of volunteers attended the Birstall Fitness Clinic in Leicestershire twice weekly for nine months, for a course of intensive physical exercise.

### Subjects and Methods

The subjects were healthy males aged 40 to 60 years who responded to publicity concerning the exercise program in the local press. Forty-seven subjects enrolled for the course and 25 of these attended regularly and completed the course. All subjects were medically examined before the first attendance.

A test battery measuring a variety of physiological, psychological and physical fitness parameters was employed prior to and on completion of the course, in order to identify changes in these parameters as a result of regular exercise.

The psychological tests included the McNair and Lorr Mood Scale and the Edwards Personal Preference Schedule. The mood scale measures the moods of tension, anger, depression, vigor, fatigue, friendliness and confusion. The Edwards test measures the tracts of achievement, deference, order, exhibition, autonomy, affiliation, intraception, succorance, dominance, abasement, nurturance, change, endurance, heterosexuality and aggression.

A non-exercising control group of 13 non-volunteer males in the same age group was similarly tested. The fact that the control group was not drawn from the same population may be seen as a criticism of the design, but it provides an interesting comparison between volunteers and non-volunteers.

## Results

The Edwards Test. It will be seen from Table 1 that the volunteers differed considerably from the population norm scores on certain traits, in particular dominance (76%) heterosexuality (64%) and achievement (61%). Low scores were recorded for deference (26%) abasement (35%) and exhibition (40%). By contrast the control group scored high on nurturance (73%) succorance (71%) and heterosexuality (61%) and low on endurance (36%) and change (40%).

Differences between the initial and final scores for individual traits were small and nonsignificant, except for the increase in exhibition in the exercise group from 40% to 53% ($p < 0.1$). However, when the traits are viewed together, the tendency for the high scores to increase and the low scores to decrease is also significant ($p < 0.05$). No such tendency appeared in the control group.

The McNair and Lorr Test. As stated previously, this test measures seven moods. Five of these moods may be described as unfavorable, namely tension, anger, depression, fatigue and confusion. The other two moods, vigor and friendliness, may be considered favorable.

As can be seen from Table 2 the mean initial scores of the exercise group were more favorable than the scores of the control group on all moods except friendliness and, surprisingly, fatigue.

For the exercise group the changes in the moods concerned at the end of the exercise course were in favorable directions with the exception of friendliness, which showed a small decrease, and depression, which remained the same. These favorable changes are signifi-

Table 1. EPPS Scores

| | | ACH | DEF | ORD | EXH | AUT | AFF | INT | SUC | DOM | ABA | NUR | CHG | END | HET | AGG |
|---|---|---|---|---|---|---|---|---|---|---|---|---|---|---|---|---|
| E | I | 61 | 26 | 51 | 40 | 51 | 41 | 58 | 47 | 76 | 35 | 46 | 55 | 59 | 64 | 57 |
| | F | 65 | 27 | 47 | 53 | 50 | 39 | 66 | 40 | 81 | 29 | 45 | 50 | 58 | 68 | 59 |
| C | I | 57 | 55 | 50 | 43 | 47 | 59 | 52 | 71 | 50 | 58 | 73 | 40 | 36 | 61 | 43 |
| | F | 45 | 61 | 54 | 48 | 40 | 50 | 54 | 75 | 39 | 43 | 69 | 36 | 50 | 70 | 36 |

Table 2. McNair and Lorr Scores

| | | Tension | Anger | Depression | Vigor | Fatigue | Friendliness | Confusion |
|---|---|---|---|---|---|---|---|---|
| E | I | 6.3 | 7.6 | 4.0 | 13.0 | 4.3 | 12.0 | 3.8 |
| | F | 5.0 | 6.1 | 4.0 | 13.5 | 3.3 | 11.6 | 2.8 |
| C | I | 6.8 | 8.8 | 5.5 | 12.3 | 4.0 | 13.8 | 5.8 |
| | F | 6.0 | 6.0 | 5.5 | 12.0 | 3.5 | 12.3 | 4.0 |

cant when taken as a whole, ($p < 0.05$). Changes in individual moods were not large enough to be significant, although it is interesting to note that the two largest changes in the exercise group were reductions in anger and tension.

Reference to the control group scores indicates that caution must be used in drawing firm conclusions from the favorable changes in the exercise group.

The control group scores showed favorable changes in four of the seven moods, namely tension, anger, fatigue and confusion and no change in depression. Such favorable changes in the control group tend to be less marked than in the exercise group with the exception of reduction of anger.

This paper is concerned with changes in psychological variables following regular exercise. No mention has been made of those volunteers who withdrew and failed to complete the course. It is perhaps worth mentioning that the initial mean mood scores of those who withdrew were less favorable on every single mood than the mean scores of the exercise group. This is highly significant ($p < 0.01$).

## Discussion

The statement "exercise is good for you" may well be true for the majority of the population where physiological health is concerned. This study has shown that individuals who volunteer to exercise are not typical members of the population, but possess a distinct personality and mood profile.

We are not in a position to compel individuals to exercise but must resort to persuasion and motivation. Exercise volunteers show small but significant changes in personality and mood as measured by the Edwards Personal Preference Schedule and the McNair and Lorr Mood Scale. The changes detected in this study may have been more significant if larger groups had been used and if the frequency of exercise had been higher. Perhaps there is an optimum level of exercise for each individual at which he benefits maximally in psychological terms and this level may not be the same as the level for maximum physiological benefit.

## Summary

Twenty-five male exercise volunteers were assessed for personality and mood prior to, and on completion of a nine months period of strenuous exercise twice weekly. Their scores were compared with a control group of non-exercising males. The exercise group presented a personality profile differing greatly from the norm in certain personality traits, scoring highest on dominance and lowest on deference. Changes in personality scores at the end of the exercise program were only marginal, but a significant tendency for the high and low scores to polarize was demonstrated. This tendency did not occur in the control group.

In the Mood test, the exercise group initially scored more favorably than the control group on all moods except friendliness. At the end of the course they demonstrated an improvement in all moods except friendliness, which decreased slightly, and depression, which remained the same. The improvements were slight, but marginally significant when taken as a whole, the greatest improvements being in tension and anger. The control group also improved four of their mood scores, but their improvements were generally less marked. It was observed that those volunteers who withdrew from the course had less favorable scores on all moods than those who completed the course.

## PART 2

### Introduction

In recent years the importance of early mobilization following myocardial infarction has been realized (Carson et al., 1973, 1976). Additionally, many centers now offer a program of physical activity as part of the cardiac rehabilitation program.

Long term preventative effects in relation to reinfarction have been demonstrated (Sanne, 1972) as a result of a sustained program of regular strenuous exercise, but the psychological state of the patients following exercise has received scant attention.

### Patients and Methods

In the autumn of 1977 a program of cardiac rehabilitation by exercise was instituted at Craigavon Area Hospital in County Armagh, Northern Ireland, as a research trial. Post-infarction male patients up to the age of 65 years were referred to the trial by the consultant cardiologist, after satisfying medical criteria of suitability for the proposed exercise program. Doctor Walsh also assumed overall responsibility for the trial.

Patients were randomly assigned to one of two groups. A battery of physiological, anthropometric, and psychological tests were applied to the patients on referral, including the IPAT Anxiety Questionnaire scale. All patients were again tested after eight weeks, and finally retested after a further eight weeks. One group, referred to as the E (early exercise) group attended for exercise in the hospital gymnasium for the first eight week period only, while the other L (late exercise) group attended during the second eight week interval only.

This double-cross-over design has certain advantages. Each patient was in an experimental group for one eight week period, and a control group for the other eight week period. No patient was deprived of the beneficial effects of rehabilitation by exercise. It also provided an opportunity to assess the relative merits of an early exercise program compared with the same program delayed by eight weeks.

The exercises were isotonic in nature, applied to large muscle groups moving through wide ranges of movement, in order to increase the demand on the cardiovascular system without causing excessive strain on any specific region of the body. Exercises included rowing, cycling, step-ups, and fast walking. The gymnasium sessions were supervised by the hospital physiotherapy staff, who ensured a sustained progression of work load at successive attendances.

## Results

The initial, intermediate, and final anxiety scores are shown in Table 3.

The reduction in anxiety scores for the two groups throughout the sixteen week period was highly significant ($p < 0.01$). Further analysis however, has not revealed any significant difference between the two groups, either during the exercise or the control periods.

The general tendency for the scores of the two groups to decrease can be seen from Table 3, but changes in the successive scores of individual patients varied considerably, some demonstrating large decreases in anxiety during the exercise period and others demonstrating increases during the same period. It has not yet been possible to account for these different patterns, although analysis of correlations with other variables measured in the study may be revealing.

Table 3. IPAT Anxiety Scores

| | | Initial | Intermediate | Final |
|---|---|---|---|---|
| E | Mean | 28.9 | 25.5 | 23.6 |
| | S.D. | 13.9 | 12.1 | 14.1 |
| L | Mean | 21.8 | 19.9 | 19.0 |
| | S.D. | 8.7 | 9.5 | 8.3 |

Summary

Twenty-four male patients who had recently suffered myocardial infarction were tested for anxiety score using the IPAT scale.

A double-cross-over experimental design was used to examine changes in anxiety as a result of rehabilitation by exercise. Reductions in anxiety scores throughout the trial were highly significant but occurred during both control and experimental situations. It was not therefore possible to conclude that anxiety reduction was a direct result of exercise. Exercise should of course continue to be used in rehabilitation because of its physiological benefits. Further work is needed to facilitate identification of those individuals who benefit psychologically from exercise.

## DISCUSSION

The protective effects of exercise following myocardial infarction have been demonstrated, but conclusive evidence of improvements in psychological variables as a direct result of exercise has not yet been demonstrated.

Part 1 of this paper showed that the personality profiles of exercise volunteers differs from the norm. It may be that those infarction patients who would volunteer for exercise would show significant reductions in anxiety, but that other patients may actually find the exercises anxiety provoking, in spite of the physiological improvements usually associated with exercise.

Part 2 of this paper has posed more questions than it has answered. It may be that some patients would benefit most from exercise rehabilitation only, while others may require a more direct psychological counseling approach (Naismith et al., 1979). Psychotropic drugs and relaxation techniques may also have an important role to play with some patients.

The problem is to devise a screening system to determine the most suitable course of treatment or combination of treatments for individual patients.

## ACKNOWLEDGEMENTS

I thank Dr. M. Walsh and the staff of the physiotherapy and ECG departments of Craigavon Hospital for the help I had from them in conducting this study. I also thank Mrs. P. McDowell of Ulster Polytechnic for her valuable secretarial help.

REFERENCES

Gelson, A. D. N., Carson, P. H. M., Tucker, H. H., Phillips, R., Clarke, M., and Oakley, G. D. G., 1976, Course of patients discharged early after myocardial infarction, Brit. Med. Jnl., 1:1555.

Hellerstein, H. K., 1974, "Rehabilitation of the Postinfarction Patient," Hospital Practice Publishing Co., Inc., New York.

Ismail, A. H., and Trachtman, L. E., 1973, Jogging and imagination, Psych. Today, 6:79.

Morris, J. N., and Crawford, M. D., 1958, Coronary heart disease and physical heart disease and physical activity of work, Brit. Med. Jnl., 2:1485.

Naismith, L. D., Robinson. J. F., Shaw, G. B., and MacIntyre, M. M. J., 1979, Psychological rehabilitation after myocardial infarction, Brit. Med. Jnl., 1:439.

Sanne, H., Elmfelt, D., and Wilhelmsen, L., 1972, "Preventative Effect of Physical Training after a Myocardial Infarction," Almqvist and Wiksell, Stockholm.

Tucker, H. H., Carson, P. H. M., Bass, N. H., Sharratt, G. P., and Stock, J. P. P., 1973, Results of early mobilization and discharge after myocardial infarction, Brit. Med. Jnl., 1:10.

# RELAXATION TRAINING IN THE TREATMENT OF ESSENTIAL HYPERTENSION

Peter Seer, Ph.D.

Rehabilitationszentrum
7812 Bad Krozingen
West Germany

## INTRODUCTION

Modern psychological treatments of essential hypertension fall into four major groups (1.) blood pressure biofeedback, (2.) relaxation training, (3.) meditation training, and (4.) approaches in which biofeedback, relaxation and meditation techniques are combined (Patel, 1977).

Most of the studies comparing blood pressure biofeedback and relaxation and meditation training are unfortunately methodologically unsound (an exception is the recent study by Blanchard, Miller, Abel, Haynes, and Wicker, 1979) and have produced equivocal results. However, based on a careful examination of non-comparative studies, it is safe to say that, in contrast to blood pressure biofeedback training, relaxation and meditation training have produced small but significant reductions in blood pressure with essential hypertensives which have been shown to persist for up to 6 months (Seer, 1979).

Blood pressure biofeedback training clearly has not fulfilled its promise. To quote from a recent review:

> Given the available data, it appears that BP feedback may simply be an inefficient method of eliciting a generalized low-arousal response (Williamson and Blanchard, 1979).

While there are at least two well-controlled studies which have found significant blood pressure reductions with progressive relaxation training (Brauer, Horlick, Nelson, Farquhar, and Agras, 1979; Taylor, Farquhar, Nelson and Agras, 1977) studies using meditation training as treatment technique have attained comparable results but were much less well controlled. In the present study which aimed at assessing the effects of concentrative meditation training on pharacologically untreated essential hypertensives an attempt was made to achieve higher methodological standards. After extensive baseline testing subjects were randomly allocated to one of three groups: (1.) meditation training, (2.) a treatment element control group, and (3.) a waiting list control group. Blood pressure was monitored over a 13-week training and a three-month follow-up period.

A further aim of the present study was to investigate the essential technique ingredients by applying a "treatment element control strategy" (Kazdin and Wilcoxon, 1976).

## METHOD

### Subjects

Forty-one essential hypertensives were selected for the present study (23 males, 18 females; mean age 43.2). None of the subjects was taking antihypertensive or psychotropic medication during the entire experiment.

### Assessment Procedures

An independent observer recorded baseline blood pressure once weekly for four weeks using a random-zero sphygmomanometer (Wright and Dore, 1970). Blood pressure was recorded in the sitting position after a standard resting period of 5 minutes. Blood pressure was taken five times at one-minute intervals and a mean value was calculated for each session. Only subjects with a mean arterial pressure of 100 mmHg or greater were included (mean arterial pressure = systolic blood pressure minus diastolic blood pressure, divided by three, plus diastolic pressure).

During the 13-week treatment/control period all subjects were scheduled for another five blood pressure assessment sessions with assessment always preceding any meditation practice. Finally, after a total of 25 weeks of meditation practice subjects participated in two final follow-up assessment sessions which were set one week apart.

### Treatments

The main experimental treatment (SRELAX, N=14) was a concentrative meditation technique which was modeled after transcendental

Table 1. Pretest, Posttest and Follow-Up Means of Systolic and Diastolic Blood Pressure (mmHg).

| | Pretest (sessions 3/4) | Posttest (sessions 8/9) | Follow-up (sessions 10/11) |
|---|---|---|---|
| | SYSTOLIC | | |
| SRELAX | 152 | 148 | 150 |
| NSRELAX | 147 | 142 | 139 |
| CONTROL | 150 | 152 | - |
| | DIASTOLIC | | |
| SRELAX | 104 | 97 | 97 |
| NSRELAX | 100 | 93 | 88 |
| CONTROL | 102 | 104 | - |

meditation (TM). However, all mystical elements and esoteric vocabulary and content were removed, and relaxation and coping are stressed instead. The technique required the subject to sit twice daily for 15-20 minutes in a relaxed position, to turn his or her attention inwards toward the effortless mental repetition of a meaningless syllable (mantra) or sound, and to return gently to this sound whenever the attention attached itself to unrelated thoughts and images. Subjects were also explicitly instructed to practice with a passive "let-it-happen" and non-analytical attitude. The major advantage of this technique over other relaxation techniques, such as progressive relaxation or autogenic training, is that it contains a detailed system of dealing with task-irrelevant mental processes which frequently occur in any given relaxation or meditation technique.

The use of a "mental device" (Benson, 1975) in our case in the form of a meaningless sound, is generally considered the most important element in concentrative meditation techniques (Naranjo and Ornstein, 1971). Therefore subjects in the treatment element control group (NSRELAX, N=14) were not instructed in the use of a sound as attentional focus but were simply taught to let thoughts go as soon as they became aware of them. Otherwise this group was closely matched with the experimental treatment in every respect.

Waiting list control subjects (CONTROL, N=13) participated in the same type and number of assessment sessions as the other two groups.

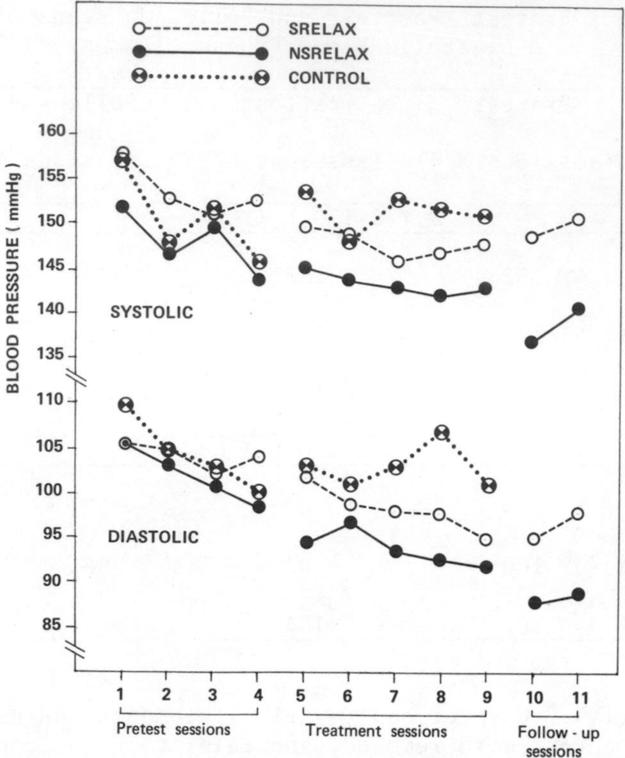


Fig. 1. Mean systolic and diastolic blood pressure (mmHg) in sessions 1 through 11 for all groups.

## RESULTS

Results were analyzed using repeated-measures analyses of variance (Winer, 1971). The results of primary interest are presented in Figure 1 and Table 1.

No significant between-group differences were found for any of the four pretest sessions. However, there was a significant within-group reduction of 7 mmHg for both systolic ($F$ (3,114)= 4.46, $p<.006$) and diastolic pressure ($F$ (3,114 = 4.10, $p<.009$) from the first to the fourth pretest session. This result stresses the importance of extended baseline testing.

After 13 weeks of training the experimental group (SRELAX) showed pretest (sessions 3 and 4 combined) to posttest (sessions 8 and 9) reductions of -4 mmHg systolic and -7 mmHg diastolic.

The treatment element control group (NSRELAX) showed comparable reductions of -5 mmHg systolic and -7 mmHg diastolic, while the waiting list control group (CONTROL) displayed a slight increase of 2 mmHg for systolic and diastolic blood pressure. However, for diastolic blood pressure only, the differences were found to be statistically significant (within-group difference: $F(1, 38) = 6.07$, $p<.02$; Session X Treatment interaction: $F(2, 38) = 3.78$, $p<.03$).

Twelve out of 14 SRELAX and 11 out of 14 NSRELAX subjects were available for follow-up testing. SRELAX subjects maintained their posttest diastolic blood pressure while NSRELAX subjects showed further reductions. However, neither between-group (t-test, two-tailed: $t = 1.94$, $df = 21$, $p<.07$) nor within-group comparisons (paired t-tests, two-tailed, for posttest-follow-up differences: $t<1$) were significant.

A different but closely related way of analyzing these data is to compare each subject's blood pressure of sessions 5-9 with his or her own pretest values (sessions 3 and 4 combined) and to express the difference in the form of percentage reduction values. The percentage reduction values for systolic blood pressure were small and nonsignificant. Percentage reduction values for diastolic blood pressure are presented in Figure 2.

They were statistically significant (between-groups difference: ($F(2, 38) = 3.30$, $p<.05$) and reached -7% in session 9 for the SRELAX, -8% for the NSRELAX and -1% for the CONTROL condition. Overall from pretest to follow-up diastolic blood pressure was reduced by 8% in the SRELAX and by 10% in the NSRELAX group.

The problem with group designs is that when large inter-individual variability in response to treatment occurs, as was the case in the present study, the "statistical treatments will average out the clinical effects" (Hersen and Barlow, 1976). If we divide our (SRELAX/NSRELAX) sample in a median split into responders and non-responders, we find in the responder group reductions in mean arterial pressure ranging from 8-17%, with a mean reduction of 12%. Diastolic pressure was clearly more responsive to treatment than systolic pressure, a finding which has also been observed in a recent study by Brauer et al. (1979) although not to such a strong degree. While before treatment 75% (N = 21) of all SRELAX and NSRELAX subjects (N = 28) had diastolic pressure of 95 mmHg and above, this percentage dropped to 43% (N = 12) at posttest and to 39% (N = 9, total N at follow-up was 23) at follow-up.

## DISCUSSION

The results of the present study clearly indicate that the mental repetition of a meditation sound was not a crucial element of the technique (see also Smith, 1976). The subjects in the NSRELAX group who were simply instructed to sit for 15-20 minutes twice a day and

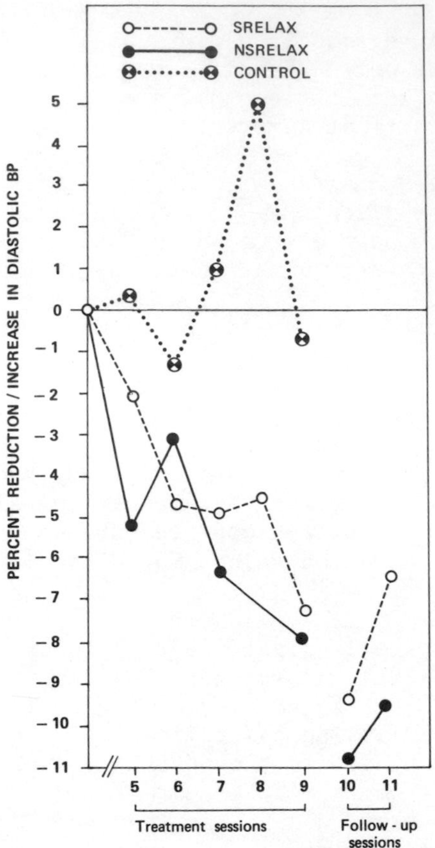


Fig. 2. Mean percentage reduction/increase in diastolic blood pressure in sessions 1 through 11 for all groups.

to let thoughts come and go, did equally well, if not slightly better, although differences between the SRELAX and the NSRELAX condition did not reach statistical significance. The question then arises, to which other elements or active components can the observed blood pressure reductions be attributed. (1.) Nonspecific treatment factors probably made some contribution. However, it is unlikely that they played a central role. Jacob, Kraemer, and Agras (1977) have demonstrated quite convincingly that, in general, placebo treatments of hypertension are significantly less effective than meditation and relaxation treatments. (2.) Interrupting one's ongoing activities twice a day and just sitting quietly in a comfortable position for a set period of time certainly appear to be important active ingredients. Various experiments have shown that even short rest periods can have marked effects on various psychophysiological parameters (Travis, Kondo and Knott, 1976; Walrath and Hamilton,

1975). (3.) A further component which to date has received little attention is the role of meditation attitude. Subjects in the present study were instructed to adopt a relaxed attitude of for example "just taking it easy and taking it as it comes", or "to not worry about how well they were performing the technique" and several others. These self-instructional sentences are implicitly rehearsed in every meditation practice and reports by subjects suggest that they tend to generalize over time to the person's natural environment.

The results of the present investigation compare favorably with other studies which also relied exclusively on one single passive relaxation or meditation technique (Benson, Rosner, Marzetta, and Klemchuck, 1974a, 1974b; Stone and DeLeo, 1976). Studies in which several techniques such as relaxation and meditation training, deep breathing, GSR and EMG feedback training and self-monitoring were combined to one treatment package have produced larger blood pressure reduction (Patel and North, 1975). Although the simultaneous application of several training procedures makes it impossible to isolate the active ingredients, these studies nevertheless suggest that a more comprehensive approach may produce better results.

Most studies investigating the psychological control of essential hypertension have been primarily sypmtom-oriented and aimed at counteracting or reducing sympathetic nervous system activity that is assumed to play a central role in essential hypertension. None of the studies, including the present one, have investigated what caused sympathetic arousal in the first place. We need to base future studies on much more sophisticated psychological and psychophysiological assessments. Patients who are referred by physicians for psychological treatment of elevated blood pressure frequently have normal resting blood pressures in the laboratory. However, there is more to essential hypertension than resting blood pressure. Blood pressure may show sharp rises in response to environmental demands. Various researchers (e.g. Henry and Cassel, 1969) have postulated that it is especially the height of the blood pressure peaks which is crucial in the development of pathological changes in the vasculature.

It is therefore suggested that in future research blood pressure should not only be taken under standard resting conditions but also before, during and after exposing subjects to relevant laboratory stressors. This would allow us to determine such important parameters as speed and magnitude of blood pressure rises and the length of time it takes for blood pressure to return to baseline levels. In addition blood pressure should be measured in real life situations, either by the experimenter or subjects themselves. Finally an attempt should be made to carefully assess the subject's idiosyncratic ways of perceiving, appraising and behavior in response to environmental demands.

Such a comprehensive approach to assessment would constitute a sound basis for a more comprehensive approach to treatment which would make use of specific behavioral techniques (Beiman, Graham, and Ciminero, 1978), and techniques of cognitive therapy and stress management. It is hoped that future research will examine the blood pressure effects of these techniques that aim at systematically teaching active coping skills and compare them with more passive techniques such as biofeedback training, and relaxation, and meditation training.

## REFERENCES

Beiman, I., Graham, L. E., and Ciminero, A. H., 1978, Setting generality of blood pressure reductions and the psychological treatment of reactive hypertension, Jnl. of Behav. Med., 1:445.

Benson, H., 1975, "The Relaxation Response," Morrow, New York.

Benson, H., Rosner, B. A., Marzetta, B. R., and Klemchuck, H. M., 1974, Decreased blood pressure in borderline hypertensive subjects who practice meditation, Jnl. of Chron. Dis., 27:163(a).

Benson, H., Rosner, B. A., Marzetta, B. R., and Klemchuck, H. M., 1974, Decreased blood pressure in pharmacologically treated hypertensive patients who regularly elicited the relaxation response, Lancet, 1:289(b).

Blanchard, E. B., Miller, S. T., Abel, G. G., Haynes, M. R., and Wicker, R., 1979, Evaluation of biofeedback in the treatment of borderline essential hypertension, Jnl. of App. Behav. Anal., 12:99.

Brauer, A. P., Horlick, L., Nelson, E., Farquhar, J. W., and Agras, W. S., 1979, Relaxation therapy for essential hypertension: A veterans administration outpatient study, Jnl. of Behav. Med., 2:21.

Henry, J. P., and Cassel, J. C., 1969, Psychosocial factors in essential hypertension: Recent epidemiologic and animal experimental evidence, Am. Jnl. of Epidem., 90:171.

Jacob, R. G., Kraemer, H. C., and Agras, W. S., 1977, Relaxation therapy in the treatment of essential hypertension, Arch. of Gen. Psychia., 34:1417.

Kazdin, A. E., and Wilcoxon, L. A., 1976, Systematic desensitization and nonspecific treatment effects: A methodological evaluation, Psy. Bul., 83:729.

Naranjo, C., and Ornstein, R. E., 1971, "On the Psychology of Meditation," Viking Press, New York.

Patel, C. H., 1977, Biofeedback-aided relaxation and meditation in the management of hypertension, Biof. and Self-Reg., 2:1.

Patel, C. H., and North, W. R. S., 1975, Randomized controlled trial of yoga and biofeedback in management of hypertension, Lancet, 2:93.

Seer, P., 1979, Psychological control of essential hypertension:

Review of the literature and methodological critique, Psy. Bul., 86:1015.

Smith, J. C., 1976, Psychotherapeutic effects of transcendental meditation with control for expectation of relief and daily sitting, Jnl. of Cons. and Clin. Psy., 44:630.

Stone, R. A., and DeLeo, J., 1976, Psychotherapeutic control of hypertension, The New Eng. Jnl. of Med., 294:80.

Taylor, C. B. Farquhar, J. W., Nelson, E., and Agras, W. S., 1977, Relaxation therapy and high blood pressure, Arch. of Gen. Psychia., 34:339.

Travis, T. A., Kondo, C. Y., and Knott, J. R., 1976, Heart rate, muscle tension, and alpha production of transcendental meditators and relaxation controls, Biof. and Self-Reg., 1:387.

Walrath, L. C., and Hamilton, D. W., 1975, Autonomic correlates of meditation and hypnosis, The Am. Jnl. of Clin. Hyp., 17:190.

Williamson, D. A., and Blanchard, E. B., 1979, Heart rate and blood pressure biofeedback: I. A review of the recent experimental literature, Biof. and Self-Reg., 4:1.

Winer, B. J., 1971, "Statistical Principles in Experimental Design", (2nd ed.), McGraw-Hill, New York.

Wright, B. M., and Dore, C. F., 1970, A random-zero sphygmomanometer, Lancet, 1:337.

# WE ALL NEED HOMEOSTASIS

P. G. F. Nixon, F.R.C.P.

Consultant Cardiologist
Charing Cross Hospital
London, England

The cardiologist deals with an extensive section of the human spectrum of disorder and catastrophe. The common conditions included in this section are:

1. GROSS UNFITNESS where small effort produces symptoms usually associated with great effort, such as forceful overactivity of the heart and heavy breathing.

2. ARRHYTHMIAS OF THE HEART, usually fast or irregular beating and dropped beats.

3. One or more of a CLUSTER OF DISORDERS which include hypertension, hyperlipidemia, hyperglycemia, increased blood coagulability, hyperuricemia and fluid retention.

4. Acute, subacute or chronic CORONARY SYNDROMES ranging from mild, infrequent and non-progressive angina pectoris to the catastrophic myocardial infarction. Usually the individual has put himself into a position where the demands upon the heart outstrip the competence of the coronary circulation at that period of his life. He has left no reserves for contingencies after a long period of exhaustion, and the disturbances of homoeostasis he brews up are harmful to the arteries. It is reasonable to believe that overwhelming demands outstrip the competence of the coronary circulation more quickly in the middle-aged than in the young, and more readily in those with severe coronary atheroma than in those without.

The currently-fashionable technically-oriented medical model is to see these cardiovascular conditions as a series of capriciously invasive "disease" processes, each, as it were, with a "life-force" of its own--a "life force" largely beyond the reach of the "possessed" individual's skill and will--requiring highly skilled and professional doctors to drive them out.

I have found this model increasingly inadequate during the last two decades, and I have come to regard it as unacceptable for four principle reasons:

1. It ignores the linkage of the cardiovascular disorders with the human disarray which precedes them.

2. It does not offer therapeutic satisfaction.

3. It does not enable individuals to grasp and follow the essential principles for recovering and defending their health.

4. It manufactures almost exclusive dependence upon doctors who haven't the time to deal with the real problems, where there should be a legitimate deployment of the numerous therapists and teachers in our midst.

I mentioned the linkage of the cardiovascular disorders with their antecedent human disarray first because I wished to emphasize our finding that the vast majority of the disorders do NOT come "out of the blue", without invitation or warning, but only after a prolonged period of human disarray. Recognizing and dealing with the disarray at an early stage is obviously the best way of preventing the cardiovascular disorders from developing, and this is the theme of my paper.

The components of the human disarray which we see as precursors of the cardiovascular disorders are:

1. A high level of behavioral arousal or excitation as judged by the amount of human effort and sedation required to produce calmness and objectivity, the essential conditions for having useful discussions about problems, for solving problems, and for adapting and habituating to fresh circumstances.

2. Deteriorating performance well below the individual's best coping ability at times of good health.

3. A behavioral pattern diagnostic of exhaustion as described below.

4. Homeostasis, already violated, or with a very fragile grip on normality.

Homeostasis is the collective name for the body's mechanisms for protecting the constancy of the internal milieu against the deformations which might be induced by changes of the world around us, and our individual reactions to them. The body has a multitude of homeostatic systems. For example, shivering protects against hypothermia and thirst against dehydration. One of the most important is the fatigue which warns us not to carry on until we are exhausted, but the programs and duties of our lives makes us selectively deaf to its voice, and our conditioning makes us scorn to listen out for it.

These four components of the disarray, namely high arousal, poor performance, exhausted behavior and homeostasis violation are also the essential ingredients of self-defeat and loss of morale. They invite defeat by difficult circumstances and difficult people.

If the current medical model is inadequate for most patients presenting with cardiovascular disorders what can be done? Quite simply we can look for a different paradigm, one that fits our observations better than the medical model, offers better therapeutic pathways, gives individuals greater power to manage things for themselves, and helps to de-professionalize and liberate the use of human therapeutic skills.

The paradigm I favor is the HUMAN FUNCTION CURVE (Figure 1) which places the various aspects of the human condition in their order of passage from healthy function to the point of breakdown (P). Arousal, behavioral arousal, describes a continuum ranging from drowsiness or unconsciousness through "normal" levels of alertness and attention to heightened states of emotional disquiet and mounting effect such as rage, alarm, terror and revulsion. Sympathoadrenal activity is usually closely related to behavioral arousal, and the catecholamine response to the challenges of every day life in some individuals approaches the levels found in phaeochromocytoma. Performance refers

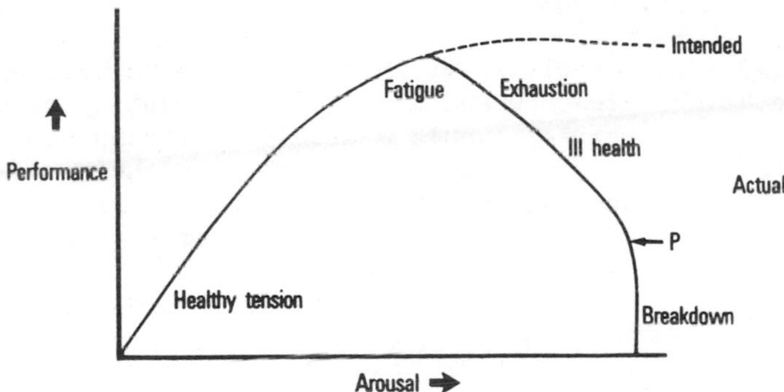


Fig. 1. Human Function Curve shows aspects of the human condition in order of passage from healthy function to point of breakdown. P equals the point at which even minimal arousal may precipitate a breakdown.

to the ability to cope with tasks. In healthy function the performance can rise to meet the demands and challenges which create arousal, demands and challenges which may come from "inside" (e.g. ambition) or from "outside" (e.g. the demands of a hard and unstable social culture). In healthy fatigue from high and prolonged arousal the performance falls off but can easily be restored by refreshing sleep. Boredom develops if there is too little stimulation and too little to do.

If high and prolonged arousal carries the individual "over the hump" and on to his down-slope many vicious circles are set up which can bring about bewildering changes in the morale, the emotions, the behavior and the health.

For example, the sleep becomes inefficient with high levels of arousal and exhaustion, and sleep deprivation tends to carry the individual down into ill-health or the point of breakdown (P). As the performance deteriorates the individual tries harder to do what is intended of him but he only succeeds in arousing himself further and aggravating the exhaustion. Fighting to close the gap between what actually can be achieved and what is intended inevitably widens it, and many people struggle on until they have induced ill-health or brought about a breakdown. The type A individuals (Friedman and Rosenman, 1974) are particularly prone to drive themselves angrily to self-destructive extremes.

The individual's position on his own human function curve can be recognized either from his external behavior or from the behavior of the internal milieu. The external behavior is more easily accessible to the observer and so I shall describe it in more detail.

## DIAGNOSIS OF HEALTHY FUNCTION

The individual feels well. His manner is relaxed and physical recreation brings pleasure and does not cause guilty reactions. Burdens and pressures that would cause loss of happiness and health are rejected. Increasing the arousal enhances the performance. Other people look upon him and his relationships as healthy and see him as adaptable and approachable. The qualities required for success, namely rapid and flexible thought, originality, vigor, expansion and capacity for sustained effort, are abundant.

## DIAGNOSIS OF ACCEPTABLE FATIGUE

The individual feels and shows reasonable fatigue, does not deny it, and takes steps to recover as soon as possible. Maladaptive habits that waste time and energy can be modified and unessential drains on the energy can be jettisoned or deferred. Performance can increase with arousal but more effort is required. Disciplined effort, youthful conditioning for competition, social pressures and mild stimulants such as coffee and cigarettes play a greater part in sustaining the performance. Sleep is adequate. Others see the individual as healthily tired but they are not made anxious because the qualities required for success are still evident. Therapy is neither sought nor required, other than reassurance that the fatigue is healthy.

## DIAGNOSIS OF EXHAUSTION

The individual commonly makes strong declarations of health and virility that are at odds with his observed behavior. He rejects the need to maintain a reasonable balance between high endeavor and relaxation, and sees no need to increase his fitness in preparation for periods of unusual effort.

Excessive burdens and pressures, disruptive of health and happiness, are accepted as inevitable because the exhaustion reduces the ability to distinguish the essential from the inessential. Increasing the arousal worsens the performance and sets up a vicious circle because widening the gap between the actual and the intended performance increases the arousal by generating anxiety and insecurity. Unrealistic views of the gap are adopted, errors increase and personal relationships deteriorate. Others can see the growth of unhealthy tension and the symptoms of strain: bad temper, continual grumbling, longer hours worked but less achieved, repeated minor sickness and preoccupation, together with insecurity, about health and the future, procrastination, losing sight of long-term aims in preoccupation with minor matters, feelings of frustration and persecution by colleagues, with complaints of lack of cooperation, technical jargon and catch-phrases replacing original thought (Kennedy, 1957).

Previously acceptable mannerisms become neurotic and disrupt peace of mind of others. Sleep becomes inadequate, increasing the exhaustion and promoting another vicious circle of deterioration. The qualities required for success disappear. The mind becomes set against change, and adaptability is lost. Leadership comes to depend upon tradition and seniority instead of ability. Eating, drinking, smoking and talking increase, and a compulsive desire for stimulating circumstances may dominate life.

Biochemical changes associated with exhaustion and a high level of arousal may be seen, such as decreases in serum iron and increases in thyroid and sympathoadrenal activity. The metabolic consequences include increases in serum cholesterol, triglycerides, uric acid, glucose, blood coagulability, heart rate and blood pressure (Carruthers, 1969; Theorell et al., 1972; Kagan and Levi, 1974; Clark et al., 1975). Fluid retention is common, particularly in women.

Attempts to bring about an improvement often make the doctor frustrated and anxious because the more severe the patient's exhaustion, the more seriously does he resist attempts to reduce his arousal. Righteous indignation and militant enthusiasm are commonly used devices which carry the arousal into ill-health. Cardiac arrhythmias, heightened awareness of the heart-beat and neurotic symptoms such as chest pain are common, and reassurance provides no more than temporary relief.

The ill-health brought about by the continuing, or increasing, arousal of the exhausted individual usually includes symptoms of sympathoadrenal overactivity. The clinical syndromes are numerous and varied, and can be seen as organic or functional according to the standpoint of the observer, and the amount of cardiovascular wear and tear already sustained by the patient. They may come to light when the patient complains of symptoms but they are often discovered when a medical examination is made annually or demanded by a spouse.

The syndromes include painless or painful cardiac disability associated with palpable and audible atrial gallop rhythm (the pre-infarction syndrome) (Nixon and Bethell, 1974), hypertension and the metabolic disorders previously mentioned. Diagnosis depends upon the clinician recognizing that the ill-health is an extension of the exhaustion; that it has adequate cause in a high-life change score, and that healthy human function is restored by treating the exhaustion and hyperarousal. It is not obtained by the exhibition of a specific remedy for a symptom, whether it be methyldopa for hypertension or coronary artery by-pass grafting for angina pectoris. Anxiety and conditioning of the individual may have removed insight, and substituted a paradoxically and blatantly illogical denial. Some individuals are incredibly tough and can continue to function in the zones of exhaustion and ill-health for years until they run out of strength or suffer a breakdown from a chance aggregation of adverse circumstances.

## BREAKDOWN IN HEALTH

Mackenzie (1908) stated that patients with angina pectoris and coronary artery sclerosis rarely presented for treatment until some distressing symptom interrupted their lives. He described the varieties of breakdown that we now call left ventricular failure, acute coronary insufficiency (intermediate coronary syndrome), cardiac infarction and sudden death. Since his day the behavior of patients and their ways of breaking down do not appear to have altered (Nixon, 1973).

Events that cause changes in the patient's customary way of life can be assessed in magnitude and duration by life-change scoring techniques, and these usually show a significant rise in the six months before infarction. There is a highly significant correlation between these life-change scores, serum uric acid level and the catecholamine output (Theorell et al., 1972). Catecholamine secretion can reach pheochromocytoma levels and cause profound changes in the blood pressure, cardiac function, blood coagulability and in the blood cholesterol, triglycerides and sugar levels (British Medical Journal, 1971; Kagan and Levi, 1974).

The common causes of high life-change scores before myocardial infarction are the same as the precursors of other forms of breakdown, and include conflicts and change at work and at home, changes in habits, frustration and defeat imposed by others, bereavement, actual or threatened loss of job and changes of work site which create housing and traveling problems.

In exhaustion and ill-health there are two main emotional responses. One is rage or frustration, and the other is insecurity with despair and hopelessness. Both are accepted as precipitants of heart failure. They probably correspond to the final common paths of fruitless activity or giving-up that are followed when the individual loses the ability to predict and maintain control over his environment (British Medical Journal, 1975). Apart from coronary illness and heart failure other forms of breakdown include hypertension and its complications, cardiac arrhythmias, gout, diabetes mellitus and hyperlipidemia. I have encountered individuals who broke down, for example, from venous thromboembolism or pyrexia of unknown origin when the problems of life became too much for them, or who avoided a breakdown by arranging a timely hernia repair or an orthopedic operation. A study of fifty consecutive patients with coronary and hypertensive vascular disease showed that the factors precipitating the breakdown were almost as numerous and varied as the patients themselves. In predicting whether an individual under hardship might break down, it is more useful to assess his reserves from his poisition and stability on his own function curve than to weigh the changes that are pressing upon him.

The individual's position on his own curve is changed whenever his arousal is increased or decreased, and extreme circumstances can increase arousal to a point at which no one can remain healthy.

The most important cause of a morbid level of arousal seems to be the threatened or actual loss of ability to understand and to control the environment and his affects highly aggressive individuals more than the passive. The commonest examples seen in cardiovascular practice are 'people-poisoning' (mind-battering, recurrent anxiety created by a person or persons whom you cannot escape), unacceptable time-pressures, high levels of resentment about changes imposed by others in hierarchies and families, and the fruitless hyperactivity responses to anxiety.

The same sort of environmental changes that cause high life-change scores before a coronary breakdown have been seen by other investigators as causing the hypertrophy of aggression (Lorenz, 1967), breakdown in managers (Kennedy, 1957), heart failure (Chambers and Reiser, 1953), and mental breakdown (Birley, 1973).

Certain deprivations, such as being a migrant or lacking an adequate support group within the community, predispose to morbid arousal (Kagan and Levi, 1974).

## DIAGNOSTIC AND THERAPEUTIC TESTING

The electrocardiogram at rest gives no information about the performance of the individual. It is a poor predictor of heart attacks even when it is taken after exercise because it is neither specific nor sensitive enough (Redwood and Epstein, 1972). The attempts to record it under conditions of intense emotional arousal may be more successful (Schiffer et al., 1976).

The coronary arteriogram provides different information about the heart but it is not a measure of the human function. It is now well known that crippling angina pectoris and severe myocardial infarction can occur in patients with normal arteriograms. It is not so well known that a middle-aged man with 99%, 95% and 80% narrowings of the three major coronary arteries can be trained to become a marathon runner (Bassler and Scaff, 1976).

In patients who have once suffered coronary ill-health or breakdown, palpation and auscultation of the chest wall over the apex of the left ventricle enable the observer to decide within a matter of moments whether the individual is shifting towards health or a breakdown. Healthier pulsations are smaller and closer to normal in area; and the fourth heart sound diminishes and merges into the first heart sound. A shift towards breakdown is marked by a larger area of left ventricular pulsation and more easily palpable and audible fourth heart sound vibrations (Bethell and Nixon, 1973; Nixon, 1974). A palpable and audible third sound gallop after a coronary breakdown (except when the patient has trained himself to become an athlete) indicates either gross left ventricular overdistension or aneurysm formation in the ventricular wall.

Of all the invasive and non-invasive techniques that are available in a modern cardiac laboratory to test for impending cardiac breakdown, I believe that the most useful are the ability to recognize the behavioral changes that mark deepening exhaustion and ill-health and the ability to detect the abnormal palpable and audible atrial sound over a distended left ventricle. The physical signs are recognized by the hand and the ear, and permanent records can be taken with the apex cardiogram and phonocardiogram (Fig. 2).

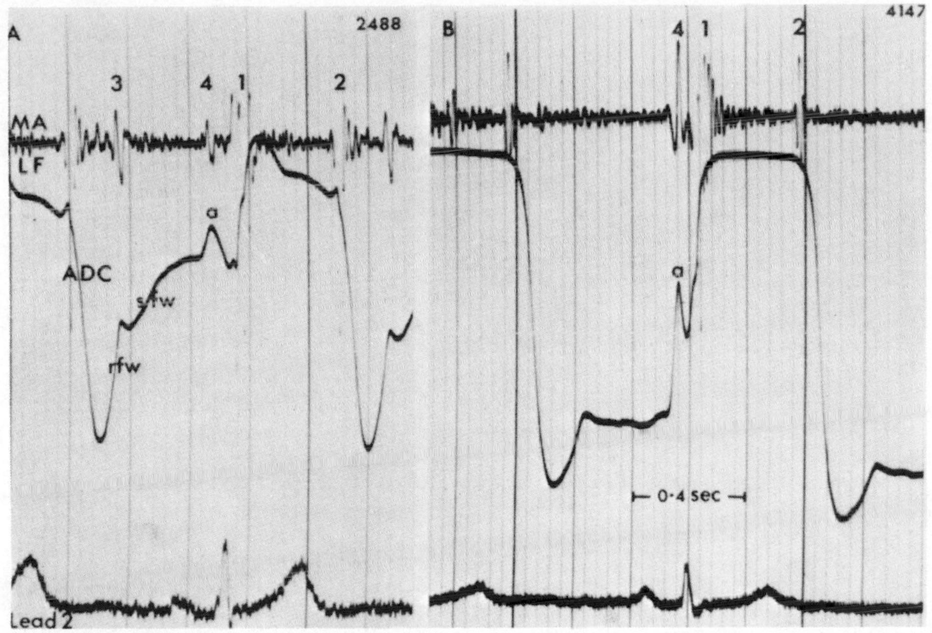


Fig. 2. (A) The normal diastolic movements and sounds displayed by simultaneous recording of the apex cardiogram (ADC), the mitral area low frequency phonocardiodiogram (MALF), and lead II of the elctrocardiogram. Diastolic filling of the ventricle occurs in three phases represented by the rapid filling wave (rfw), the slow filling wave (sfw), and the small 'a' wave caused by atrial systole. (B) The abnormal diastolic movements and sounds in a patient with ischaemic heart disease. The rapid filling wave is attenuated while the 'a' wave is exaggerated and is accompanied by a loud atrial sound (4). (Reproduced by courtesy of the Editor, British Heart Journal, 1973, 35:229).

Hospital care and investigation can be alarming and expensive, and the arousal caused by admission can precipitate a breakdown. In most cases of raised blood pressure, angina pectoris, hyperlipidemia and hyperuricemia it is reasonable for the family doctor to carry out the first diagnostic and therapeutic test by removing exhaustion and morbid arousal at home. The patient may then be returned to work at a rate which does not re-exhaust him and recreate the ill-health.

## SURVIVAL TACTICS

Survival tactics include any maneuver which helps an individual to achieve and maintain his best level of performance to minimize his risk of defeat by exhaustion, ill-health or breakdown and to diminish the likelihood of premature aging of his arteries.

Obvious requirements are:

1. An awareness of position on the human function curve.

2. An awareness of the possibility of shifting the position on the curve in a better direction, even in the face of apparently hopeless circumstances.

3. The will and the discipline to achieve a desirable shift.

4. Skill in simple tactics for managing arousal and exhaustion before they take too deep a bite.

People who become ill or break down with cardiovascular conditions usually have made four serious errors and they should be aware of them:

1. They have ignored the rule that men are not designed to function indefinitely under unremitting and maximal effort--periods of intense workload must be balanced with phases of relaxation.

2. They have failed to get an adequate amount and quality of sleep.

3. They have failed to keep themselves fit and tough enough for their chosen life-styles.

4. They have failed to realize that sheer will-power cannot overcome exhaustion and ill-health; only 'boxing clever' can buy time for recovery.

Thus while it may take a considerable amount of will-power to leave the action and go away to'recharge the batteries' when exhaustion is beginning to bite, it is essential to do so before the vicious circle of exhaustion can take hold and destroy the ability to cope.

The tactics necessarily include methods for reducing arousal, or obtaining relaxation in the midst of circumstances conducive to excessive arousal. The skilled masseuse is a particularly effective teacher, perhaps because she is permitted to touch and because her ability to induce relaxation provides a pleasant experience which the individual can soon learn to reproduce for himself.

It is important to know how to avoid sleep deprivation. When sleep deprivation is prevented it is difficult for an individual to fall into violation of homeostasis or self-defeating behavioral patterns.

It is also important to know how to train the patient who has suffered from cardiovascular disorders to become fit enough and tough enough to do what he wants in life without falling into the ever diminishing and vicious cycles of excessive arousal, exhaustion and defeat. He must stay on the upslope while he learns how to raise his human function curve to an adequate height. Once the tactics have been learned, many patients who have suffered even from multiple myocardial infarction enjoy training themselves to high levels of fitness: we have runners and skiers, but we do not go to the point of producing marathon runners like my friend Terry Kavanagh in Toronto (Kavanagh, 1976).

Sir John Hackett understood the natural therapeutic processes very well indeed when he wrote "I had gone into battle as fit as a prizefighter and certainly owed to this reserve of physical strength much of the resistance I had been able to offer to the stresses of the last few weeks. There was not now much left to draw on. I was soon to fall so low that it would take much time and care to creep back up again," (Hackett, 1977).

Unfortunately, we have been passing through an era of medicine in which logic and commonsense have sometimes been displaced by the pharmaceutists' propaganda which urges little more than the removal of symptoms with drugs. However, it does not take much nous to see, for example, that bringing down the blood pressure with a drug is not the same as removing exhaustion and the smell of defeat. Inhibiting the heart's responses with a betablocker such as propanolol is not the same as dealing with frustration, exhaustion and despair. The heart is an interesting organ: it hasn't a telephone line to tell consciousness when it has been used badly for too long, and it tends to complain with pain when it has been ill-used to a dangerous degree. I am glad to say that the ability to silence this voice with drugs and operations is not yet universally accepted as a high point of medical progress.

In my consulting practice most of the people carrying the labels of hypertension or coronary disease can achieve healthy function if they learn how to be rid of hyper-arousal, exhaustion and sleep deprivation. A great advance is made if they are taught nothing more than to be still sometimes, and to cultivate a healthy respect for fatigue.

## REFERENCES

Bassler, T. and Scaff, J., 1976, Impending heart attacks, Lancet, 1:544.

Bethell, H. J. N., and Nixon, P. G. F., 1973, Understanding the atrial sound, Brit. Heart Jnl., 35:229.

Birley, J. L. T., 1973, The effect of the environment on the individual, Proc. Roy. Soc. Med., 66:96.

Brit. Med. Jnl., 1971, Editorial: The murmuring heart, 4:125.

Brit. Med. Jnl., 1975, Editorial: Response to stress and ulcers, 2:458.

Carruthers, M. E., 1969, Aggression and atheroma, Lancet, 2:1170.

Chambers, W. N., and Reiser, M. F., 1953, Emotional stress in the precipitation of congestive heart failure, Psychosom. Med., 15:38.

Clark, D. A., Arnold, E. L., Foulds, E. L., Brown, D. M., Eastmead, D. R., and Parry, E. M., 1975, Serum urate and cholesterol levels in Air Force cadets, Aviat. Space Envir. Med., 46: 1044.

Friedman, M., and Rosenman, R. H., 1941, "Type A Behaviour And Your Heart," Wildwood House, London.

Hackett, J., 1977, "I Was A Stranger," Chatto and Windus, London.

Kagan, A. R., and Levi, L., 1974, Health and environment--psychosocial stimuli: a review, Soc. Sci. Med., 8:225.

Kavanagh, T., 1976, "Heart Attack? Counter Attack!", Van Nostrand Reinhold, Toronto.

Kennedy, A., 1957, Individual reactions to change as seen in senior management in industry, Lancet, 1:261.

Lorenz, K., 1967, "On Aggression," Methuen and Co. Ltd., London.

Mackenzie, J., 1908, "Diseases of the Heart and Aorta," Oxford Medical Publications, London.

Nixon, P. G. F., 1972a, Recovery from coronary illness, Rehab., 81:23.

Nixon, P. G. F., 1972b, Rehabilitation of the coronary patient, Physio., 58:336.

Nixon, P. G. F., 1973, Coronary heart disease and its emergencies, Pract., 211:5.

Nixon, P. G. F., 1974, Non-invasive techniques in angina pectoris, in: "Angina Pectoris," O. Paul, ed., Medcom Press, New York.

Nixon, P. G. F., and Bethell, H. J. N., 1974, Preinfarction ill health, Am. Jnl. Cardiol., 33:446.

Nixon, P. G. F., Carruthers, M. E., Taylor, D. J. E., Bethell, H. J. N., and Grabau, W., 1976, British pilot study of exercise therapy II patients with cardiovascular disorders, Brit. Jnl. Sports Med., 10:54.

Redwood, D. R., and Epstein, S. E., 1972, Uses and limitations of stress testing in the evaluation of ischaemic heart disease, Circ., 46:1115.

Schiffer, F., Hartley, L. H., Schulman, C. L., 1976, Am. Jnl. Cardiol., 37:41.

Theorell, T., Lind, E., Froberg, J., Karlsson, C., and Levi, L., 1972, A longitudinal study of 21 subjects with coronary heart disease: life changes, catecholamine excretion and related biochemical reactions, Psychosom. Med., 34:505.

AUTHOR'S NOTE

Portions of this paper are extracted from "The Human Function Curve," Practitioner, 1976, Vol. 217, pp. 765 and 935, published by Practitioner, London, and "The B.M.A. Book of Executive Health," 1979, Chapter 5, published by Times Books, Ltd., London. Permission to reprint is granted by the publishers.

# PAIN AND TENSION CONTROL

# DIAGNOSIS AND TREATMENT OF MYOFASCIAL PAIN ARISING FROM TRIGGER POINTS

John Mennell, M.D.

Professor of Physical Medicine (Retired)
University of California at Davis
Vero Beach, Florida

Dr. Rinehart has correctly told us (see "Tension and Stress," this volume) that stress is the reaction of the body to noxious stimuli. He has given us a fairly comprehensive list of such stimuli which we face in our every day lives. Whether tension is the cause or a result of stress remains moot. The adverse reaction of the person to noxious stimuli, however, is largely predictable in its effects which are manifested in the musculoskeletal system, the various visceral systems and in mental changes.

But in every presentation which we have heard so far there is a singular lack of reference to PAIN as a cause of stress and tension. Though some of the noxious stimuli are obviously associated with pain, certainly not all of them are. No one has yet addressed themselves to the possibility that stress and tension in themselves are causes of pain which must be relieved before stress and tension can be controlled.

It is fairly well accepted that psychological therapy fails to bring relief of psychological problems arising from chronic pain when there is an underlying cause of pain which is unrecognized, ignored or untreated. Some authorities admit that as much as 40% of psychiatric illness has an organic cause. For these two reasons we should always be searching for common causes of pain which afflict our patients and to which but scant attention may have been paid in the medical literature.

Today too much attention is being paid to developing adaptive therapies for patients with chronic pain rather than towards the prevention of it by better diagnosis and treatment of acute pain.

My presentation is confined to two little-recognized but very common causes of pain in the largest of the body systems -- the musculoskeletal system. Afflictions of this system are probably the least well understood of any to which man is heir. Yet musculoskeletal pain and/or dysfunction are the commonest complaints which bring patients to the physician's office.

The first condition I wish to mention is synovial joint dysfunction which is a mechanical cause of pain. It has three etiological factors -- intrinsic trauma, immobilization (which includes disuse and aging) and it invariably follows the resolution of any more serious pathological condition affecting directly or indirectly any other part or structure in the musculoskeletal system. Rightly your program committee discouraged detailed exploration of this common condition because, unless you can learn to diagnose it (which takes a minimum of 20 hours) you cannot learn how to treat it at a meeting of this kind. So however well the subject may be presented, you would have nothing useful to take home with you after the meeting is over.

But I would draw your attention to your national societies of manual medicine (manipulation) and/or therapists with whom you should be able to study and develop your interest in the subject when you get home.

The second condition I shall discuss at length. It is the irritable myofascial trigger point. Most of our knowledge about trigger points we owe to Dr. Janet G. Travell and for the most part my presentation reflects her original work.

The irritable trigger point as a diagnosis of a cause of pain has received scant recognition in clinical medicine. Yet it is an extremely common cause of both acute and chronic pain and of disability which may be of recent origin or of very long standing.

Muscle spasm or guarding may be a prelude to the development of irritable trigger points and irritable trigger points cannot really be present in muscle without spasm resulting. Unrelieved spasm results in muscle shortening and Starling's Law tells us that a short muscle is a weak muscle and a long muscle is a strong muscle. So part of the trigger point syndrome is weakness not necessarily associated with atrophy and with restriction of some voluntary movement.

At this point I wish to digress from considerations of diagnosis to consideration of treatment of an irritable trigger point. Successfully to treat a trigger point which is causing pain, it is necessary passively to stretch the involved muscle so that it may resume it normal resting length and then to strengthen it by using lengthening exercises. Most therapists use shortening exercises which, in this instance may well aggravate the patient's condition.

## DIAGNOSIS

The diagnosis of an irritable trigger point is largely based on recognizing the pattern of pain which a patient describes as being typical for a trigger point in any given muscle. These patterns of pain bear no relationship to any neuroanatomical distribution. They bear no relationship to patterns of radiating pain nor pain from neuritis or entrapment syndromes.

## PREDICTABILITY OF LOCATION OF TRIGGER POINT

Yet given a pattern of pain you can predictably locate the source of it in a specific place in a specific muscle by palpation. The patient is not aware of the location of the source of pain. In other words, the source is silent with regards to pain insofar as the patient's awareness goes. However, on palpation the source is locally tender and irritation of it by palpation sets off the predictable pattern of pain or makes it worse.

On palpation of the trigger point there is a ropey feeling in the muscle which is well localized, and palpation produces a twitch within the muscle which Dr. Travell calls the "jump sign". This has nothing to do with the patient jumping in response to the pain which palpation produces. The location of the trigger point in any given muscle is the same in the same muscle from patient to patient; and the pattern of pain from any given trigger point is also the same from patient to patient.

## PREDICTABILITY OF PATTERN OF PAIN

The recognition of the pattern of pain is the main clue to the diagnosis, and the source, being in a predictable place which, on stimulation, predictably reproduces the pattern of referred pain, which is also predictable, clinches it. Then, the results of treatment, if properly applied, are also predictable. Pain is relieved, and this is lasting so long as the cause of the irritable trigger point has been relieved also.

Because muscles learn bad habits quickly and unlearn them very slowly, if at all, symptoms even of very long standing arising from hitherto unrecognized trigger points may be relieved quite readily.

The trigger point syndrome is a clinical syndrome and it is only recently that the so-called "scientific method" has led research to uncover "facts" to support the clinical hypothesis. Electromyography and study of biopsy material under the electron microscope have shown predictable even if rather non-specific changes in areas of muscle where trigger points clinically lie. Medical research usually eventually supports the findings of clinical research especially when clinical findings are so predictable. Meanwhile patients should not be denied treatment that works for lack of so-called scientific support of that work.

## ILLUSTRATIONS OF PAIN PATTERNS

To illustrate the patterns of pain predictably arising from trigger points, I have chosen the common trigger points found is some of the head and neck muscles. They are Dr. Travell's patterns of pain and are reproduced by permission. In each picture "x" marks the location of the trigger point. The black areas are the locations of pain of which a patient invariably complains. The darker stippled areas indicate places where the patient often complains of pain and the lighter stippled areas indicate areas where the patient may sometimes complain of pain. In the head and neck the patient may complain of pain on the side of the head opposite the side of the trigger point. It should also be noted that we are not only talking of superficial pain or muscle pain but also of deep bone pain and pain deep in the ear. When tooth pain is involved, the teeth may also be sensitive to pressure and changes of temperatures.

## ETIOLOGY

To complete the diagnostic picture of the irritable trigger point which causes pain which should make the entity more acceptable to those who look askance at clinical work which is unsupported by "scientific fact", we must look at the etiological factors which cause trigger point irritability.

---

Fig. 1. The illustration shows trigger points indicated by an "x" in certain muscles of the head and neck. Black areas indicate where the patient invariably complains of pain. The dark stippled areas indicate where the patient frequently complains of pain. The light stippled areas indicate areas where the patient sometimes complains of pain. Copyright by McGraw-Hill, 1952. Travell, Janet, and Rinzler, Seymour. "The Myofascial Genesis of Pain." Postgraduate Medicine, May, 1972, Vol. 11:425. Reprinted by permission of the publisher and Dr. Travell.

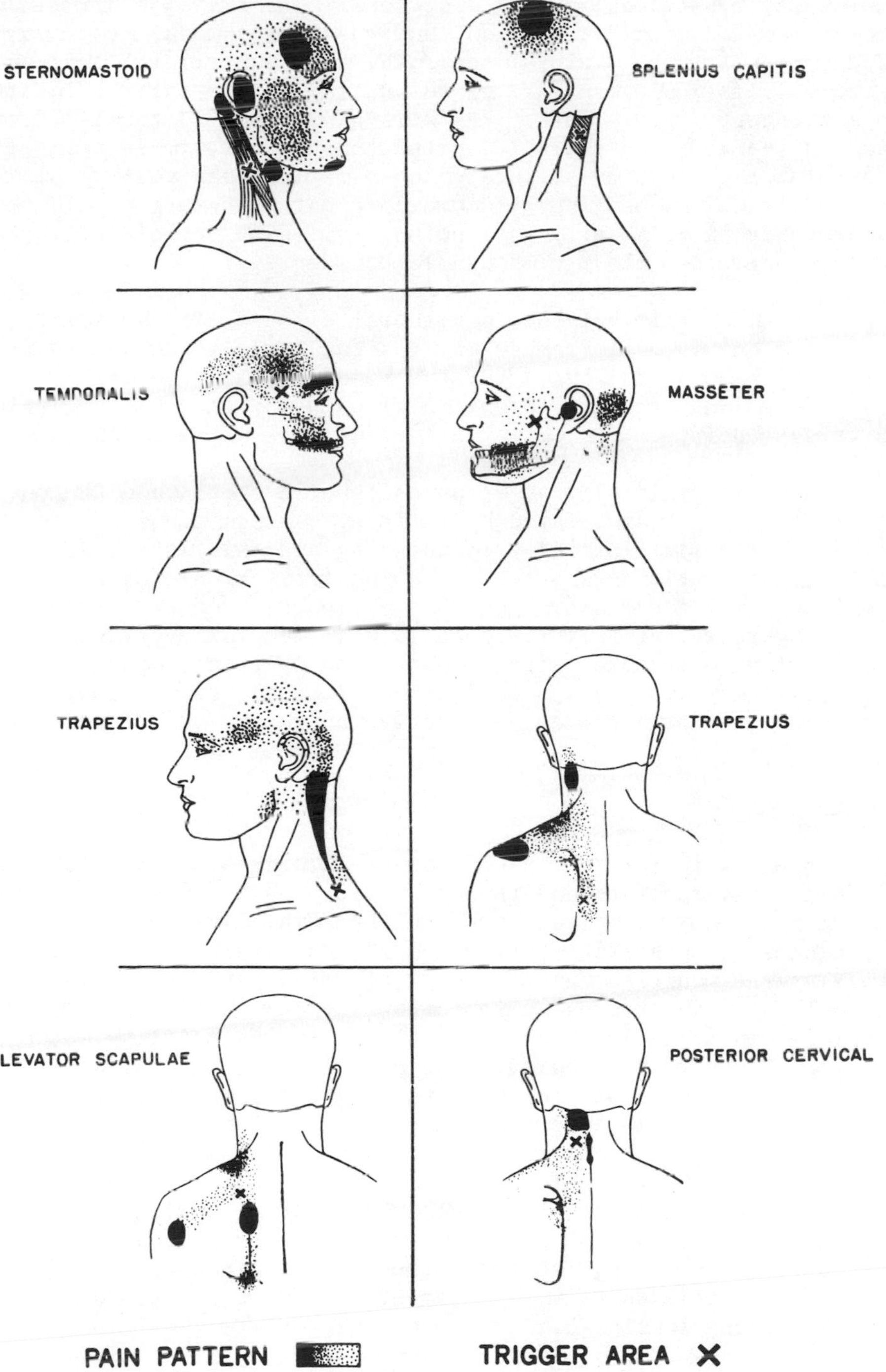
STERNOMASTOID
SPLENIUS CAPITIS
TEMPORALIS
MASSETER
TRAPEZIUS
TRAPEZIUS
LEVATOR SCAPULAE
POSTERIOR CERVICAL
PAIN PATTERN
TRIGGER AREA ×

Causes my be local to the musculoskeletal system and include such things as muscle contusion, and muscle spasm, be it primary of due to guarding. Painful scars, be they superficial or deep, especially following surgery or burns, may be the initial insults to activate trigger points. Bad work habits and postural defects such as the long leg-short leg situation or just simple painful feet, in an attempt to relieve which a patient abnormally shifts his body's weight bearing. Innumerable patients suffer pain from unrecognized irritable trigger points following personal injuries in automobile and other compensable accidents.

Causes may initially be in visceral disease and the somatic component of visceral disease may residually leave an active trigger point which persists long after the resolution of the disease. Neurological and vascular problems of pain may also be the irriators of trigger points.

Causes may initially be of psychosomatic origin and the muscle involvement may be initiated by fatigue, stress, tension, fear or anxiety. The list seemingly is unending and this is one reason why working with patients who are suffering from chronic pain is so time consuming and requires unusual patience. But when this is rewarded by relief of pain it is so much better for everyone concerned than having to teach a patient adaptation by transcutaneous nerve stimulation, biofeedback, acupuncture, hypnotic suggestion, escalating drug therapy and even destructive neurosurgical procedures.

## THERAPY

There are two primary therapeutic approaches to extinguish irritable trigger points and thus to relieve pain. One is non-invasive using a vapocoolant spray on the skin. This employs the principles of counterirritation and the results can be explained by applying the modified "gate theory" of Melzak and Wall. The second approach is invasive, using injection therapy. Dr. Travell uses ½% procaine in physiological saline. It is the needling which "explodes" the trigger point. The procaine has a local anesthetic effect, of course, but probably its most important feature is that it has a curare-like effect which enhances relaxation of the muscle into which it is introduced.

The common denominator of both therapeutic approaches is relaxation which is achieved, as Dr. Travell says, by disconnecting the muscle from its message center. Then the muscle does not know what to do, so it relaxes. At that moment it can be stretched to its normal resting length which is a pain-free state.

The Muscle Stretch

The success of either treatment appears to depend on the stretching of the muscle applied passively by the therapist either during the application of the spray or immediately after the procaine injection. It is essential for the patient to maintain a normal resting length whilst restoration therapy is undertaken. This involves the application of gentle heat to the muscle and gentle lengthening exercises with graduated resistance together with rest from function of the sick muscle while healing is taking place. Intermittent use of the spray and stretch usually has to be applied also. Whichever method of treatment is used, the skillfulness of the therapist cannot be underestimated in its importance. Both methods have to be learned in a painstaking way. This fact is surprising to many as both techniques look so easy when they are demonstrated.

## REASONS FOR THERAPEUTIC FAILURES

Later you will be given an opportunity to view my film which Dr. Travell made with me demonstrating the techniques we use when treating patients with irritable trigger points using the vapocoolant spray.* We demonstrate a minor variation of technique when treating painful muscle spasm or myostatic spasm. I anticipate your agreement that it all looks so easy. We have a few bottles of spray here. After you have watched the film, try it. Then I anticipate your agreement that it is not so easy.

So, the first reason of failure in treatment, if your diagnosis is correct, is lack of familiarity with the technique of treatment using the vapocoolant spray. In this area of technique, using too much spray on the skin and chilling the underlying muscle makes the patient worse. And, by the same token, overstretching the muscle being treated makes the patient worse.

When part of the symptom complex being treated has a radicular or neuritic basis, stretching the muscle also stretches the inflamed nerve and the patient's pain worsens. In this instance the spray is a diagnostic tool. The same thing may be said of the spray when the cuse of painful muscle spasm is guarding a joint from painful movement when joint instability is caused by ligament laxity or tear or rupture. When the spray overcomes the spasm and at least part of the pain, as it does, the patient's symptom of pain recurs and is worsened immediately when activity is resumed.

---

*Film distributor: Richard Lambert, P. O. Box 701, Stinson Beach, California, 94970. Vapocoolant spray: "Fluori-Methane"; Gebauer Chemical Co., Cleveland, Ohio, 44104.

If there is an active trigger point or painful muscle spasm in a muscle following fracture-healing in a long bone associated with loss of bone length then the muscle can only be stretched to an adapted resting length. This militates against successful treatment. Similarly aseptic necrosis or other such condition affecting a long bone, resulting in bone shortening, makes it difficult to relieve pain from spasm or a trigger point. Stump pain in amputees often falls into this category. Such pain is often mistaken for neuroma pain which surgery fails to correct.

Sometimes the cause of spasm or an irritable trigger point may have been overlooked and not eradicated. Then, even though it is possible to relieve the pain temporarily, it is readily reactivated. Quite frequently this occurs when the cause of spasm is joint dysfunction to which I made reference at the beginning of this paper. And in this context we must go back to general medicine and search for and correct if present any nutritional deficiencies and rule out the presence of such things as gout, hypothyroidism and subclinical rheumatic diseases.

Another cause of failure of vapocoolant spray therapy is when the therapist treats a satellite trigger point(s), overlooking the parent one. All trigger points must be treated, and patterns of pain often overlap. The parent one is the most important one, however. And when a trigger point is a manifestation of the somatic component of visceral disease, treatment of the primary disease is the important thing in the management of the patient's pain.

Please, then, remember as you watch the film which briefly touches on the probable reasons why the vapocoolant spray relieves myofascial pain and muscle spasm, that it is essentially a means of teaching how to use the spray and how to stretch various muscles to their normal resting length.

The film may give the impression that one application of the spray or one treatment session achieves the relief of symptoms. Sometimes one treatment is enough to relieve the patient of pain permanently. Most often, however, a course of therapy is required and several treatment sessions are needed. Retraining muscles and strengthening them so that painless function may be resumed may take several weeks as mentioned earlier. Sometimes the spray fails to extinguish a trigger point even when properly used; then injection of the trigger point may have to be undertaken initially.

## INJECTION THERAPY

As most of you may not use injection therapy I am confining my remarks to the reason for failure of a form of treatment which should succeed. In a way they are similar to the causes of failure using the vapocoolant spray.

Dry needling is as successful as needling with a local anesthetic and, parenthetically, this may be one explanation for the success sometimes achieved by acupuncture. But the needle must be inserted into the trigger point very accurately. Bleeding must not occur. Blood around the needle point in the trigger point or in the area immediately surrounding it, further irritates the trigger point and pain persists. The same thing happens if any injection fluid is used in amounts in excess of ½ cc. Puddling of fluid in and around a trigger point stretches the tissue and further irritates the trigger point.

Dr. Travell specifically recommends the use of procaine because of its curare-like action which possibly produces more profound relaxation of the muscle being treated. Steroids should not be added to the injection fluid because they increase the volume of fluid injected unnecessarily and also because they may crystalize out at the injection site thereby reactivating the trigger point by physical irritation. No epineherine should be used because vascular changes in the trigger point may be a source of irritation.

Even if injection therapy relieves pain, this is only a start of a treatment management program which has been outlined above.

## SUMMARY

As you all know, the name of the "new therapeutic game" is "pain clinic". Alas in almost all of these clinics there is an ignorance of two very common causes of pain in the musculoskeletal system to which patients should not have to adapt because they are diagnosable and curable. In stress and tension control centers, synovial joint dysfunction and irritable trigger points must be recognized and can be treated with predictable relief of pain. These clinical entities must be ruled out before any thought is given to adaptation therapy. Stress and tension can only be relieved or controlled imperfectly unless all physical causes of pain have been removed.

# HOLISTIC STRATEGIES IN THE MANAGEMENT OF CHRONIC PAIN

Durand F. Jacobs, Ph.D.

Chief, Psychology Service
Pettis Memorial Veterans Hospital
Professor of Psychiatry
Loma Linda University Medical School
Loma Linda, California

## INTRODUCTION

Years of faulty problem definition have added significantly to the ranks of 40 million chronic pain sufferers in the United States. The isomorphic conviction that persistent pain complaints must be based on some underlying organic pathology has led well-meaning clinicians inadvertently to incur drug addiction, to surgically augment pain, to foster functional invalidism and to further dislocate the lives of chronic pain sufferers and their families. The economic toll of lost wages, medical costs and related expenses, and compensation payments is estimated to be as high as 35 to 50 billion dollars a year. The extent of mismanagement of chronic pain patients has reached the proportion of a national tragedy.

The author described the "Chronic Pain Personality Syndrome", a particularly disabling reaction to chronic pain which is highly resistive to treatment. The syndrome is comprised of a tightly knit set of learned behaviors directed to defending the patient against the phobic-like fear that his level of pain may worsen. Over a period of time these behaviors pervade and reshape the entire lifestyle of the sufferer. The marked resistiveness of the syndrome to treatment is attributed to the pattern of interactions that have evolved over a number of years between the identified patient, his significant others and selective features of his environment.

Holistic Strategies in the Management of Chronic Pain

This paper analyzes the onset, course and prognosis of the syndrome. Some diagnostic aids are offered to facilitate early identification of this syndrome among more typical reactions to acute and chronic pain.

Certain similarities are drawn between this particular type of chronic pain patient and the alcoholic, including the conditions that must prevail before either is amenable to treatment aimed at learning more adaptive coping methods within an altered life style.

## DEFINITION

The Chronic Pain Personality Syndrome (CPPS) is defined as "an integrated set of pain-related behaviors acquired through experience by a injured person to reduce his apprehension that his perceived level of pain may worsen".

The syndrome refers to public, observable, potentially measureable behaviors. The term "injured" is used in the generic sense of tissue damage, loss of function, impaired soundness or hurt due to disease, illness or trauma. The "integrated set of pain-related behaviors" include four classes of behavior: (a.) verbal complaints or reports of subjective pain states, including discriptions of autonomic nervous system reactions, (b.) expressive behaviors such as grimacing, wincing, grinding of teeth, clinching of hands, doubling up, twitching, etc.; (c.) body positioning that serves to "guard" or "armor" the site of pain from kinesthetic or external stimulation. The above three classes of behaviors in turn are presented as justification for a fourth type: consequenting behaviors. Consequenting behaviors vary with circumstance and setting, but generally disengage the injured person from a variety of self-care, social, sexual, interpersonal, occupational, and recreational pursuits. The overall complex of behaviors that constitute the syndrome for a given individual are "integrated" in the sense that they are internally consistent and mutually supportive. In the aggregate they serve to communicate both the presence and the consequences of injury, pain, disability and handicap.

The Chronic Pain Personality Syndrome is best understood as a generalized adaptive response to a perceived stress condition. While appearing stable in the short term, a detailed history will reveal that the behaviors comprising the present syndrome had gradually evolved from a series of reciprocal interactions between the patient, his significant others and selective features of his environment. Over time some pain-related behaviors may have been added, while others may have been replaced or modified into their present form within the syndrome. Nonetheless, a highly individualized sub-set of coping behaviors can be seen to persist throughout the period of time that the individual has complained of his particular pain condition. These will be consistent with enduring features of the person's environment and with characteristic modes of stress management shown by the individual in the past. The person showing a CPPS will attempt to consolidate and freeze his physical surroundings, interactions and general life style so as to exercise maximum control over them, and to reduce the likelihood of unexpected disruptions in the elaborate defenses he has constructed against increased pain.

When circumstances beyond his control significantly change the pattern of interaction between the patient and his physical or social environment, one may expect a corresponding accommodation in the behaviors comprising the CPPS.

## AIDS TO DIFFERENTIAL DIAGNOSIS

What behaviors permit the clinician to discriminate between patients with acute or extended pain complaints and those who may be developing a Chronic Pain Personality Syndrome?

Pain is a subjective experience involving the complex interplay of three tenses: present pain, remembered pain, and expected pain.

Erickson and Rossi (1979) have noted that: "Nothing so much intensifies pain as the fear that it will be present on the morrow. It is likewise increased by the realization that the same or similar pain was experienced in the past... This and the immediate pain render the future even more threatening."

Most pain patients focus their complaints on recent past or present sensory or functional difficulties. However, the potential CPPS patient appears unusually preoccupied with avoiding anticipated pain. When carefully examined, one notes that the behaviors that comprise the syndrome are less in response to present or past experienced pain, but serve mainly as a pre-emptive and defensive mobilization against expected future pain. Consequently, the ratio between respondent vs. anticipatory pain-related behaviors demonstrated by a patient often can alert the clinician that an acute or extended pain episode may be developing into a Chronic Pain Personality Syndrome.

The clinician also can expect the range, frequency, and intensity of direct pain complaints and pain-related behaviors in the acute and extended pain patient to diminish during the process of active treatment, recuperation and stabilization following injury. On the other hand, direct pain complaints and, particularly, consequenting behaviors will tend to persist and become elaborated over time in the potential CPPS.

Another index may serve to identify the patient with a CPPS. This is the sheer number of non pain-related activities engaged in during a typical day or week. Acute pain patients will show a gradual increase in the sum of their post-injury activities involving self-care, socialization, occupational pursuits, recreation, etc. The post-injury course for the potential CPPS patient will be one of progressively reduced activities. Parenthetically, increase in gross activity level is the best single index of improvement for any pain patient. Indeed, the central strategy in holistic approaches to pain reduction is one of stimulating and maintaining ever-enhanced levels of self-determined, self-controlled and participatory activities of every stripe.

A key factor for distinguishing among persons with acute pain and extended pain conditions and the potential CPPS is the relative levels of optomism/pessimism they reflect when contemplating future pain. Persons suffering acute pain expect it to diminish over time. Those with extended pain conditions will anticipate good days and bad days around a stable mean. The potential CPPS patients expect that their present level of pain will remain high and likely increase. Consequently, depressive features (and sometimes anger) are more prevalent in the latter group.

The acute and extended pain patient is not comforted if what he does (or what others do for him) produces no reduction in his immediate perceived level of pain. In contrast, the CPPS patient is comforted after he (or those involved with him) complete actions to avoid future pain. (In this context "comforted" refers to a measurable lessening in the generalized level of muscle tension secondary to localized pain complaints.)

The CPPS patient is observed to relax almost immediately after action is taken which he believes will prevent his experiencing increased pain. This generalized relaxation response occurs much more rapidly than could be expected from direct action of the chosen drug or other intervention. Thus, it is the avoidance act, itself, which reduces the patient's anxiety and its structural and physiological concomitants. This convert drama is overlooked by the patient (and many clinicians) who attribute the visible resultant effects of reduced discomfort wholly to the action of the injection, pill, or other intervention. As a result, the patient's tendency to make use of avoidant methods is strengthened, as is his conviction that to do otherwise is to court disaster.

Close questioning will reveal that the patient has not empirically tested the efficacy of his avoidant behavior. That is, to see if failure to exercise the avoidant procedure would actually result in his experiencing increased pain. Thus, a pattern of superstitious behavior is established and elaborated, maintained by the false and unvalidated belief that to do otherwise would produce dire consequences. Through this mechanism the CPPS tends to expand like a series of concentric barricades, each serving to remove the person even further from expected (but never experienced) sources of greater pain. Unfortunately, while the patient continues to avoid experiences that he sincerely believes may incur increased pain, he progressively removes himself from interactions with the world around him, eventually approaching a condition of social isolation, static tension and inactivity.

One is impressed by the similarity between those exhibiting a Chronic Pain Personality Syndrome and persons showing phobic reactions.

Like other phobias, the CPPS may be seen as a special form of fear which:

(1.) is out of proportion to the demands of the situation;
(2.) cannot be explained or reasoned away;
(3.) is beyond voluntary control; and
(4.) leads to avoidance of the feared situation (Marks, 1969).

The special fear of the CPPS patient is of anticipated pain, not a remembered kind or amount of pain, but an unknown open-ended pain, possibly of overwhelming proportions. It is these elements of uncertainty, uncontrollability and potential catastrophe in the anticipated event which begin to explain the urgency, desperation and panic shown by certain pain patients when they are delayed or blocked from following their established (preventative) treatment regimens.

## DEVELOPMENT OF THE CPPS

Let us now examine the development of the CPPS in greater detail with reference to:

(a.) its onset
(b.) its course
(c.) its prognosis, and
(d.) its response to holistic treatment strategies.

### Onset

The onset of the CPPS is usually gradual and insidious with fragmented sequences of pain-related behaviors being superimposed on direct somatic complaints. Behaviors characteristic of the CPPS come to dominate direct somatic complaints three to six months after the occurence of the precipitating injury or illness. The physician should consider a psychological consultation when, despite accepted medical interventions, specific (and especially non-specific and non-localized) pain complaints persist beyond the expected course of recovery for the particular condition.

## Course

The course tends to follow a three stage progression:

Stage 1. Response to Acute Pain. This is the immediate post-injury period, lasting as long as three to six months. It is a time of active treatments to reduce the injury and the pain associated with it. During this stage virtually all patients are passive and receptive to actions taken by health care providers. Being in crisis, they are highly suggestible and quick to agree to medical, surgical, orthopedic and pharmocologic procedures proposed as remedial for the injury or palliative for the pain. They perceive treatment as a necessary but disruptive intrusion in their usual mix of daily activities. Pain management is seen as the sole responsibility of the physician and totally outside the patient's direct control. This stage is analogous to stage one (emergency reaction) in Selye's "general adaptation syndrome." (1974).

Stage 2. Attempts at Self-control of Chronic Pain. Those whose pain did not respond to treatment in Stage 1 join the ranks of the millions of chronic pain sufferers. This stage opens with the growing realization that past and current treatment attempts to relieve their pain are not succeeding. Persons in transition between Stages 1 and 2 will be seen to "shop around" for new physicians and surgeons, including those willing to try more radical methods. Major geographic moves to what is hoped to be a more agreeable climate sometimes occur, along with changes to work settings believed to be less aggravating to the pain condition. As new circumstances and still more therapists fail to relieve the pain, the patient's quest becomes more frantic. He begins to seek more exotic sources of possible relief outside the established health system. After many failed interventions, the patient becomes resigned to having a chronic pain problem. His strategy becomes one of "how best to live with the residual pain" and also "how to keep it from getting worse". This connotes a major shift from seeking other-directed remedies to one of self-directed attempts at pain management.

## A Brief Disgression

The tendency of health professions to lump all chronic pain patients together has contributed to the delay in identifying the

CPPS.

By far the greater number of persons who suffer continued pain learn to accommodate it and usually to subordinate it in pursuing their life goals. For purposes of comparison in this paper, these are termed "persons with extended pain".

Those who have been identified as showing the CPPS constitute a minority of all persons suffering pain. For a variety of reasons not fully understood, the CPPS patient subordinates other life goals to a singular, extended, compulsive search for pain-lessening and pain-avoiding methods. During Stage 2, the "person in extended pain" and the CPPS patient show the following radically different responses to their respective conditions of continued pain:

Persons in extended pain. They live in hope that some new surgical procedure, or drug or gifted practitioner may one day save them. They view their pain as entirely physical in nature and continue to look to the organized health delivery system for ultimate relief. Meanwhile, they proceed to make those accommodations in their personal self-care, work, family and social activities which permit them to approximate previous levels of functioning as best they can despite a fluctuating but continuing state of perceived pain. The goal of this group is to salvage and maintain as much of their pre-injury life style as they can, supported by treatment regimens designed to limit the negative consequences of pain in their day to day activities. These treatment regimens ordinarily include some combination of moderate exercise, heat and whirlpool, weight control, use of prosthetics and occasional non-narcotic drug use. Such persons characteristically report that "keeping occupied", physically and mentally, serves to temporarily distract them from experiencing pain. Overt complaints of subjective pain tend to stabilize or lessen, expressive behaviors such as grimaces tend to disappear; body positioning stances become less dramatic and more localized. "Consequenting behaviors" which serve to disengage the person from activities of living are actively avoided. Medical assistance is sought sparingly, and usually at times of particularly acute flare-ups. Pharmaceutical drug use is usually restricted to aspirin or substitute products and muscle relaxants. Alcohol (or soft drugs among younger patients) may be used epsodically to obtain their analgesic or soporific effects.

The emergence of the CPPS. An unknown proportion of the total continued pain population (perhaps one in seven) proceeds to develop a full blown CPPS. Several distinguishing features appear to mark the entry of the CPPS group into a radically new life style justified by past injury and dominated by phobic-like avoidance of possible pain-enhancing situations. Unlike the relatively passive, philosophically accepting extended pain patient, the CPPS group assumes a demanding, often belligerent and sometimes adversarial stance towards physicians and the health care system. Their interaction with the health care system is more manipulative than supplicant. When seen by the primary health provider the CPPS patient has a ready list of somatic complaints and claims of creeping invalidism (including requests for the physician to document his plight for insurance, retirement or legal applications). Close to the top of the patient's demands are those for more and/or different pain medications, modifications or additions to prosthetic devices, evaluation for surgery or other exotic interventions. Sooner or later complaints and recriminations against the present or former care provider or "the system" will be made because of their failures to provide relief to the sufferer. In time the patient will overutilize and exhaust the resources and patience of the primary care provider to the point of becoming an unwanted burden. At this time treatment is terminated or the patient is referred for "psychological" help or to a pain clinic.

During Stage 2 the CPPS group show increasing evidence of magical thinking about the power of certain medications, behavioral rituals, favorite prosthetics, even the presence of other people in preventing the pain from getting worse.

Their range of daily activities contracts and becomes increasingly stereotyped. This is fueled by anxiety that pain may increase if one's rigidly scheduled activities are altered. Any previous resistance to taking narcotic or tranquilizing drugs rapidly disappears and is replaced with a growing dependency on an increasing number of them. Well-meaning physicians may compound the polypharmacy, since patients seldom agree to eliminate a previous pain medication when adding a new one.

Gradually, the person's life becomes dominated by pain-related behaviors devoted to the containment of present pain and the avoidance of anticipated pain. The frantic, disorganized reaching out for relief in all directions which characterized their entry into Stage 2 is eventually replaced by a tightly-structured, obsessive-compulsive "game plan" focused on defending against anticipated pain. The state of continued generalized tension engendered by this behavior drains the individual of energy, lowers his irritability threshold, blunts his motivation to participate in non-pain related activities, and progressively diminishes his involvement in other life roles such as work, school, social life, recreation, personal interrelationships and even self-care activities.

The patient's attempts to deal with his present level of pain and to avoid additional expected pain exacts an awesome toll on his physical, mental, emotional and economic resources, (as well as those of other persons in his family circle). Nonetheless, this state of affairs typically continues for many years. Throughout this stage the individual remains convinced that his condition is wholly physical in nature. He will agrily reject any suggestion that he might profit from psychological assistance. Overtures by exasperated physicians and family members to involve the patient with such resources or refer him to formal pain programs are rarely successful. Any suggestion that the cause of his present discomforture may be other than physical threatens the integrity of his entire defense system and all that has been invested in it.

His belief system, energies and adjustive behaviors have become so sharply focused on the avoidance of future pain that strategies offered to reduce his present generalized tension state are relegated to secondary importance. Forceful attempts from without to deprieve him of his medications and their deleterious side effects or alter his other defenses against anticipated pain are met with extreme anxiety, anger and panic. Thus, the patient remains locked in a self-defeating and basicly unproductive course of action which not only affords him little relief from experienced pain, but may even worsen it. His only recompense lies in his deep personal conviction that short of such actions, his pain would have gotten even worse. This stage is analogous to stage 2 (resistance to stress) in Selye's "general adaptation syndrome".

Stage 3. Exhaustion. Stage 3 often begins precipitously with the patient suddenly admitting that his own and other's attempts to cope with his actual and anticipated pain either have failed or can no longer be maintained. The patient is disabused of the power he had invested in his drugs, protective devices and behavioral rituals. He is mentally, physically and emotionally exhausted, and has lost hope of being able to carry on much longer. Typically, his income is insufficient for personal maintenance, he has acquired large medical bills and he is deeply in debt. Often the supportive folk system that had been manipulated to sustain him has eroded or fled. The patient perceives himself as about to fall into his own personal labyrinth of most awful imagined fears. At this juncture the patient's anxiety and frustration may drive him to extreme actions against himself or others. The risk of acting out becomes more critical as the patient sees himself as about to be abandoned.

During this period of extreme crisis, the patient is once again open to professional help. He has no energy to resist and little left to lose. With his defensive system in disarray, he again becomes highly suggestible and amenable to relinquishing control of his life to others. This stage is analogous to the final stage (exhaustion) in Selye's "general adaptation syndrome".

The progression of the CPPS patient through the above process is reminiscent of the stages of alcoholism described by Jellinak (1960) and Tiebout (1953). Unfortunately, it is beyond the scope of this paper to pursue the many striking similarities that exist between persons who have developed the CPPS and those who have developed a pattern of chronic alcoholism. Indeed, the two syndromes often coexist in the same patient.

PROGNOSIS

Patients referred to pain programs are usually seen years after the precipitating injury or illness.

By this time they can be expected to have had two or more surgeries and spent many thousands of dollars on their condition. They will in all likelihood be dependent or frankly addicted to several drugs, unemployed, broke and receiving some type of aid and attendance from family or public agency. Some will be doggedly seeking some form of financial compensation for their condition.

They are typically angry and bitter about the health care system which has not only failed them, but now has rejected them as unsuitable for further physical or pharmacologic interventions. They resist and resent the implication that the source of their pain complaints is "in their heads". They tend to see themselves as "victims" rather than petitioners of the health care system.

Once the CPPS has become full blown (i.e., midway in Stage 2) the prognosis for psychotherapy or as a pain program candidate is extremely poor until the patient has reached Stage 3. Most patients referred to pain programs while showing behavior patterns described under Stage 2 can be expected to reject the program or leave it after a few days. The few that remain longer will likely become disruptive or otherwise attempt to sabotage the program from within. Rarely will such patients complete a pain program and, if they do, their farewell to staff likely will be in the form of a brickbat accusation that they were mistreated, harangued and, certainly not helped.

However, the prognosis in a pain program becomes very positive once the CPPS patient is willing to admit: (a.) that all that he and others have done has not been sufficient to reduce or prevent his pain, (b.) that his life has become unmanageable; (c.) that his is powerless to carry on; (d.) that he is willing to give up his medications and prosthetics as requested; (e.) that he is ready to surrender himself fully and unconditionally to a new kind of psychosocial treatment program, and (f.) that his family (or significant other) supports and is willing to participate actively in the program. As more of these conditions prevail, the better the outlook becomes for breaking the patient's pattern of self-defeating behaviors.

Much has been published in recent years about the rationale, program and results of various pain centers (Sternbach 1974; Newman et. al, 1978; Fordyce, 1976). All report some measure of success through application of a combination of techniques including desensatization and reconditioning, guided relaxation with or without biofeedback, controlled exercise, self-hypnosis, extensive educational offerings on stress and body functioning, group discussion, etc. Most pain programs have multidisciplinary staffs trained to address the multifaceted behavioral, social, economic, vocational, cognitive, sensory, physiologic, philosophical and spiritual aspects of the patient's life that have become casualties of the chronic pain syndrome. Packaged in various forms these programs all represent an holistic approach to chronic pain problems.

The programs that appear to provide the best outcomes offer a total, extremely active inpatient therapeutic environment where a group of pain patients are retained for three to six weeks.

This removes the patient from the network of counter-productive involvements in his home environment, while providing a total substitute designed for unlearning pain-related behaviors and acquiring new and more effective coping skills. With support and encouragement from staff and patients with similar problems the program member joins in an intensive regimen of acquiring relevant self-knowledge, self-confidence in his own self-control capabilities and a sense of personal accountability for the apparent vagaries in his pain experiences and general welfare. Better results have been observed when significant others are actively involved as frequent visitors and scheduled participants in the residential program, and where a three to six month follow-up is maintained through group meetings with former patients and their families.

In designing rehabilitation programs for chronic pain patients one cannot help but be impressed by the utility and direct applicability of programs and methods developed for the rehabilitation of alcoholics, including the recent development of Pain Anonymous Groups.

At present there are approximately three hundred pain clinics and residential pain treatment centers in the United States. Many of these will be instrumental in leading patients with CPPS from anguish and despair to a second chance at a happier life.

## REFERENCES

Erickson, M. H., and Rossi, E. L., 1979, "Hypnotherapy: An Exploratory Casebook," Irvington Publishing Inc., New York.

Fordyce, W. E., 1976, "Behavioral Methods for Chronic Pain and

Illness," Mosby, St. Louis.
Jellinek, E. M., 1960, "The Disease Concept of Alcoholism," Hillhouse, New Haven.
Marks, I. M., 1969, "Fears and Phobias," Academic Press, New York.
Newmann, R. L., Painter, J. R., Seres, J. L., 1978, A therapeutic milieu for chronic mental patients, Jnl. Hum. Stress, 4:8.
Selye, H., 1974, "Stress Without Distress," J. B. Lippincott, New York.
Sternbach, R. A., 1974, "Pain Patients: Traits and Treatments," Academic Press, New York.
Tiebout, H. M., 1953, Surrender vs. compliance in theraphy with special reference to alcoholism, Quar. Jnl. Stud. on Alcohol, 14:58.

# TENSION IN DENTISTRY

# EVOLUTIONARY INCREASE IN INTELLIGENCE AND THE PERCEPTION OF STRESS IN DENTISTRY

Kevin J. Lewis, B.D.S.(Lond.), L.D.S., R.C.S.(Eng.)

General Dental Practitioner
Department of Conservative Dentistry
London Hospital Dental School
London, England

The appearance of that much-favored term "uptight" in recent years lends weight to the popular suggestion that modern man is under greater stress today than ever before. Phrases such as "the hustle-bustle of the city" or "hassle" or "pressure of work" and "the stress of modern life" encourage our self-indulgent belief that we are scaling greater heights of stress endurance than our predecessors, and so comfortable are we in this presumption that we do not pause to question its validity.

Throughout time, stress of one kind or another has afflicted every living thing. Man is merely the latest development in a long evolutionary history, and is distinguished primarily by the development of intellect. My belief is that this evolutionary increase in intelligence has conferred mixed blessings.

Survival is, of course, the most essential and fundamental function of any living thing. To enable any living organism to survive, some adaptation must be possible whereby adverse life conditions can be overcome. In plant life, this is seen in the storage of food reserves in bulbs and tubers so that the lean winter months can be more easily survived, or again in the way in which root systems extend and deepen in periods of drought, in an attempt to secure water.

In other words, a living unit must be able to adapt itself to a change of circumstances. A gradual change of circumstances requires a gradual process of adaptation; a sudden change demands an immediate adaptive response. Failure in this respect may mean death, and it is through successful adaptation that the survival of the fittest has taken place in the evolutionary process.

Let us consider briefly those threats to survival which face lower animals, and which demand adaptation. Many attempts have been made to categorize both the threats themselves and the response, but in its simplest form let us consider them as primal stresses; i.e., those which have been present since life began.

1. The threat of confict
2. The threat of food deprivation
3. Threatened environment

1. The Threat of Conflict: For most animals this implies the threat of a (usually mortal) combat with a rival animal or predator. The threat is, of course, of the conflict itself and the possibility of injury, pain or even death. It was upon this situation that Walter Cannon based his "fight or flight" hypothesis of stress response.

2. The Threat of Food Deprivation: The need to engineer one's own survival through adequate food supplies is inborn. Only much later comes an awareness of the need to provide for one's dependents as well as for oneself, and although in lower animals this may be instinctive, in man it is usually a conscious, reasoned decision made in the face of emotional and social pressures.

3. Threatened environment: This could mean loss of habitat (the destruction of a bird's nest, or sudden deprivation of habitat such as faces filed mice annually at harvest time). It could also imply a change in environmental status and/or hierarchy, for example the arrival of a new lion in the lair to compete for the attentions of a lioness. Birds and bees alike violently resist any attempted invasion of their nest/hive. So do badgers, rabbits and so on. Many birds are noted for their territorial behavior and this is in resonse to a true, primal stress. (It is the same primal stress for man in some extreme situations such as faced by earthquake or flood victims. The stress accompanying this kind of natural disaster is immediately evident, and takes the form of an unanswered question: "Will I be able to survive this disaster?" or more succinctly, Will I die?" In such extreme circumstances, the individual usually has no previous experiences of this nature to draw upon, and no firm answer is possible.

While the question remains unanswered the stress remains, for the stress is embodied in the uncertainty. Once the crisis has passed the individual can say "I have survived" and a second flood or earthquake will be less stressful in as much as the individual can recall the successful survival of the first episode.

If these, then, are the primal stresses, how and why do we respond to threats that do not fall into these categories? As has been said, the lower animals respond instinctively to potential threats: the snake coils, the cat's fur bristles and so on. The primal stresses often represent a life-or-death situation, and it is appropriate that the body has developed a system of response equal to the dramatic and instantaneous nature of some situations.

Indeed, throughout evolution, those species that were able to refine their perception of stress and to improve the quality and efficiency of their adaptive response were able not only to improve their own chances of survival, but through natural selection have endowed successive evolutionary generations with an increasing facility to adapt in a changing world. Species who could not or would not adapt have become extinct.

The chameleon has adapted by the extraordinary ability to change his skin color, making him less vulnerable to predators. The amphibious frog demonstrates his remarkable response to the environmental demands that have been made upon him, as if to emphasize the enormity of his achievement in coping with both land and water conditions.

Man has been in existence for a brief, almost imperceptible span compared to the millenia since life first appeared on earth. Yet our arrogance is astonishing if we believe that our survival is somehow "guaranteed" whereas many thousands of other species have already become extinct. There is no doubt that we, too, must engineer the survival of our own species by adapting to modern-day threats. Otherwise we, too, will become extinct--possibly by nuclear holocaust (another example of how our increased intelligence has led us perilously close to disaster), or by otherwise polluting the very environment upon which we depend for our existence. Perhaps, indeed, it will prove to be stress-induced disease that brings about the undoing of the human race. Certainly, we should take careful note of the evidence of successful adaption as exemplified by all the animals around us, and resolve to develop our own adaptive facilities accordingly.

Although we dental surgeons at least no longer have a daily fight for survival against hunger, thirst or predators, although we no longer have to build primitive shelters against the elements, we still believe that the stresses which we are currently experiencing in our practice lives are far greater than those primal stresses met by our evolutionary ancestors. How can this be so?

Basically, man's evolutionary increase in intelligence has enabled him to perceive stress in ever more varied and numerous situations; some people have a diminished capacity for adaptation and feel threatened by situations which others would see as trivial and innocuous. Some individuals may have a double-edged problem in that not only do they perceive stress in more areas than their colleagues, but their facility for successful adaptation may be undeveloped or absent.

The evolutionary process of natural selection will continue to favor those who can distinguish between the situation which really does constitute a genuine threat in one way or another (i.e., a true primal stress) and the situation which merely represents a minor challenge, an obstacle to be overcome -- the everyday stimulus which is beneficial in that it helps to develop the adaptive response of the individual to changing life circumstances.

A realistic and discerning approach to the perception of stress can only come through autogenic training. I realized soon after entering dentistry that this was a "sink or swim" situation. I experienced that tightness, that "keyed-up" feeling that was quite different from the pleasurable stress I enjoyed on the rugby field. After a few months of genral practice, I began to appreciate that there were simply too many potential stressors to respond to in general practice, and I could not expect my body physiology to continue to respond to them all without some kind of protest.

When I first graduated as a dental surgeon, suffused with what I like to describe as youth, energy and enthusiasm, I remember vividly arriving at my first meeting of my local British Dental Association branch. It was a depressing and harrowing experience indeed to survey the ranks of battle-weary colleagues, faces either drawn and ashen with fatigue or flushed with the hypertensive effects of their latest intra-oral campaign. They exchanged tales of such anguish, trauma and harrassment that it remains a source of wonderment to me that dentistry is still my chosen profession. But why dentists? What singles them out from other professional colleagues such as solicitors or accountants?

Friedman and Rosenman observed that you could always recognize the dentists at a party by the way they would look anxiously-- and unconsciously-- at their watches at intervals of three minutes or so throughout the evening. The "famous last words" of a dentist are said to be "give me more time-- I need more time"!

The time factor is certainly a major source of stress. The busy National Health Service practitioner will schedule from 20 to 100 patients per day. Each booked appointment time is a deadline in itself and throughout the treatment of each patient the spectre of the next deadline looms closer with the passing of each minute. The pressure of time is almost universally perceived as stressful and it is quite commonplace for a dentist in NHS practice to be anything from 30 minutes to an hour late at some point in the day.

Another enormous problem for the NHS dentist is decision-making, (the piece de resistance of my friend and colleague Dr. Jim Dyce). The dentist is continually faced with clinical decisions since each appointment represents a practical exercise which must terminate with a high-quality end product. He is attempting to fabricate restorations as intricate as any jeweler, and the fine control and manual dexterity demanded of him in some procedures is exceptionally high. and yet his work cannot be carried out under the ideal conditions of a workbench; the dentist must operate in a very confined area in which the conditions are continually changing. Cheeks, tongue and lips all combine to sabotage his painstaking efforts, and the continual flow of saliva into the working area is a further complication. Some areas of the mouth are extremely difficult to illuminate successfully, adding to the problems of access and visibility.

The high-speed turbines that are the tools of his trade are furnished with diamond cutting instruments which are small but extremely potent. At several thousand RMP, the patient's lips, tongue and cheeks all need protection. This may also limit access and visibility. The equipment must be water-cooled and the working area is continually sprayed with a fine mist of pressurized water, which must be evacuated by high-volume suction, another item of equipment to be accommodated in what was a limited working area to begin with.

The atmosphere in which he works contains a bacteria-laden aerosol which is further loaded with mercury vapor whenever amalgam fillings are inserted or removed, and residual anesthetic gases may be an additional problem. The noise levels both with the high-speed turbine, ultrasonic scaling equipment and high-volume suction are very high for a large part of the day and he may be exposed to x-ray radiation every day of his working life. His working posture in the days when the dentist worked standing up was astonishingly bad. Even with modern, supine or "low-seated" dentistry, very few surgeons adopt a balanced operating position. Of course, some of these hazards can be eliminatee by taking appropriate and effective precautions but they are no less real.

At every stage in the creation of a final restoration, further decisions are required to update the restorative plan for the teeth in question, to select the correct materials for the procedure in hand, and so on.

Throughout these procedures, the patient may be apprehensive, his perioral musculature tense and he may have difficulty in swallowing or breathing which may or may not be psychological is origin. All these nonverbal signals of distress are communicated to the dentist who must nevertheless remain reassuring and sympathetic, although such problems are hardly making his own task any easier.

All this is repeated for every patient in the day, and not only must these procedures be carried out "against the clock", but the added pressure arises in the NHS that the dentist is remunerated directly on a piecework basis -- the less he produces, the less income he recieves. It is hardly surprising that performance satisfaction and frustration figure largely in the dentist's problems. The more self-critical dentist is continually dissatisfied with the level of his performance, and others simply drop their standards of self-expectation and may even take pride in their ever increasing quantity rather than quality of output. In this way their ego can be salvaged from an otherwise impossible situation.

There are then various areas of interpersonal conflict between the dentists and (a.) the patient, (b.) his dental nurse and other chairside staff (c.) his reception staff and those responsible for the flow of patients into and out of his surgery (d.) his laboratory technicians (e.) his professional colleagues, partners or employees, (f.) his suppliers and other trading associates.

The dentist has at one moment to be both surgeon and businessman. He has the economic pressures to maintain a viable business and adequate personal income. He may have the conflicts of partnership or the frustrations of being an associate with little or no say in the running of the practice. He may be an employer with all the problems associated with employee legislation and industrial tribunals.

His is not a retail but a production industry. He therefore has equipment which can, and frequently does, break down. Almost every breakdown in a dental practice requires immediate attention if treatment is to continue. He is similarly dependent upon dental materials of a specialized nature.

When Meyer Friedman and Ray Rosenman described the Type A personality, I wonder if they realized how accurately they were describing the archetypal British dentist working within the NHS.

The typical NHS dentist over-schedules himself and inevitably runs late for his appointments. Frantically, he "goes into overdrive" working faster and faster and hopefully becomes less and less late for each subsequent patient. What he will not do, of course, is concede that he will have to do less than he had intended for one or more patients in order to return to schedule again. Such a suggestion is, of course, anathema to a Type A, who assesses his own performance in terms of quantity of achievement.

Nurses who cannot mix materials, pack amalgam carriers, pick up and pass instruments, load syringes, write up notes, etc., as quickly as the Type A himself are a great source of frustration. So also is the patient who enters the surgery and begins a five-minute ritual of coat folding, lipstick removal, collection of vast quantities of Kleenex from the depths of an enormous handbang, extensive search for the special case for her glasses, etc.

"What do you mean, we've run out of amalgam, nurse?" bellows the irate Type A at his cowering assistant. While still placing the lining in the cavity he demands that the amalgam be mixed while considering a suitable punishment for his wayward employee and making a mental note to telephone his supplier for more amalgam before seeing his next patient-- polyphasic activity in the extreme.

With all these frustrations, our Type A is now running very late indeed, and as if this wasn't enough, the next patient is ushered in red-faced and steaming. You've guessed it. He, too, is Type A, understandably furious and frustrated that his long wait has prevented him from matching his own targets of high achievements for the day. Nothing, of course, arouses the aggressive and/or hostile feelings of the Type A subject more quickly than another Type A in full flow. We are all set for a bloodless conflict, much to the detriment of both parties.

None of these sources of stress I have described above could really, however, be considered as primal stresses. None represent a life-or-death situation. The dentist knows that, just as he overcame all these pressures yesterday and the day before, so also will he overcome them today and tomorrow.

What the dentist must do, therefore, is to learn to distinguish and differentiate between the challenges that really are important and those which are not. He must learn to delegate as much of his decision-making as possible to others. In short, he must learn to control his <u>perception</u> of stress as it appears in his everyday life, to minimize his <u>exposure</u> to potentially stressful situations through better management, and to learn to control his <u>response</u>. But first he must take the time to learn about stress itself.

We may have come a long way from our evolutionary ancestors, but we still have a mighty long way to go. Successful control of stress is a process of continual learning, and it is to this end that we are all gathered to this unique international conference.

# DECISION-MAKING: THE MOST RELEVANT RESEARCH OF OUR TIME

James M. Dyce, D.D.S(Penn.), L.R.C.P.(Edin.), L.D.S. (Glas.)

Dental Surgeon
London, England

## INTRODUCTION

In this paper we will examine a process which is as commonplace as breathing. Yet is is "the most relevant research of our time".

It is "decision-making".

Breathing starts at the first slap on the stern by the helpful midwife. Decision-making is a very close second activity. At the first arrival in the world - is it joy or shock? - the "foetus plus three seconds" lets out a howl. Everyone is relieved and delighted. The baby has made a decision to react. How may decisions did it make about life while in utero? Much time could be spent in discussion of the evidence on this!

Twenty, thirty, forty years later, experience has added a cautionary measure to our decision-making.

One developing skill involves the long-range view we take of our personal future. We decided today in the best interest of tomorrow's future - as we see it. We may plan to get to the top (whatever that means), or to leave behind social conditions of our personal upbringing, or to gain name, fame or fortune.

## DERAILMENT

Such plans have already set a path which derails us from participation in the evolutionary process. To repeat, we have already derailed ourselves from participating in the evolutionary process.

We have become irrelevant to the needs of the future.

I have put it as strongly as that because my purpose is to raise with you the need at this time for new thinking. By "new" I mean "new" - not as the soap advertisements go in television commercials: "whiter than white".

We have been derailed by a presumption about our vision for ourselves.

Of course we may know what we want to be. We may set out to carve our way through the conditions of our environment. Yet our plans for ourselves may take little account of the speed of change in our environment. That change outpaces all our current updating lectures, seminars, graduate study degrees. These primarily aim to provoke man's imagination to invent new techniques, new materials. They have very little to do with the real needs of the world.

We still become overtaken by events. We may resign ourselves to this and puff along behind. Or we may believe it is up to us to design events. The second makes the stress-story rewarding.

## TO WHAT ARE WE RESPONDING?

The question we are looking at in this paper is: "To what are we responding?"

Being notoriously ill-informed and ill-equipped in business affairs, we design systems for six-handed dentistry, which takes us further away from the one-to-one relationship with the patient.

The needs of production, and economic gymnastics, constantly overlay our thinking. How much of this is reaction to someone else's plan for the economics of the country? How much does it deal with the ideas which we see shifting the thinking of millions in the headlines or on the media? There is an immense gap in our thinking here, a gap which needs contemplation. It has gone almost unexamined throughout the entire century-and-a-half of the organized teaching of dentistry.

Without such contemplation, we take no account at all of the constructive part we can, and ought to, play in the evolutionary growth of man on this planet.

A FORWARD LEAP

Everyone is aware of the microprocessing revolution today. The phrase comes easily off the tip of the tongue. Not so readily do we foresee the real implications of this forward leap and its effects on human beings. In Britain it is only now that we assess the human effect of the Industrial Revolution as we observe the 150 years since the end of the first phase.

The workaholics produce machines with very exciting delivery systems. We, who are concerned for the treatment of stress disorders, are beginning to read the signs of the mixture of accelerating life patterns. We sense the serious trial confronting our Western political system. Few are aware of the ideological revolution. There is confusion as to what this means. We are aware of the claiming of rights by groups at all levels of society, and the certainty of future high unemployment, etc. The uncertainty of employment is less likely to apply to us in the "stress business" because we are in a sellers' market. Nowadays more people are more worried. More people expect to have more health service delivered to them on an "almost free" basis. Our Royal Commission on the Health Service, whose work has just been completed, is to recommend that this service should be entirely free of charge to the patient.

So far, I have yet to see any prior condition that the patient should "mend his ways", change his habits. That would be difficult to legislate.

Once again we will drift into social schemata which offer well-intentioned hand-outs without facing up to personal disciplines. This must produce more confusion because men are ill-equipped to read the consequences. But venture into this area of the consequences of our ideas we must.

The very first sentence of the leading article in the British Medical Journal of July 28, 1979, states: "We can easily spend the whole of the Gross National Product". The Royal Commission on the National Health Service had no difficulty in believing this proposition on financing put to it by one medical witness.

Of course there is just a vague global sum of money available, not the GNP. So, who is to get the money? Who is to be deprived of money?

In one sentence we have moved out of technology, clinical practice, into the dilemma of success surrounding us.

## SO WHAT OF THE PHILOSOPHY OF PRACTICE?

I understand that in the U.S.A., undergraduate medical schedules include the subject: "Perspectives in Medicine". This begins to reestablish that lost subject: "Philosophy". Philosophy used to be taught to medical personnel. But, at the time of the Renaissance, man decided he was clever enough and need no longer ask questions about the meaning of life or God. Before then, philosophical questions ranged around the field where God mattered. Men sought an ideology then.

The swing of the pendulum in the United States, away from grading students with A,B,C, towards labelling them as "satisfactory" or "unsatisfactory" was, I understand, an attempt to decrease anxiety and increase creative study. It was an effort to let people develop as they wished without first establishing the basic disciplines and penalties. It exhibited the flaw in decision-making which takes no account of human nature in the raw.

## LIMITED LIABILITY SCHOLARSHIP

People respond to the need for survival. It evokes competition. We have yet to turn this survival instinct into a fascinating, creative exercise primarily concerned with the survival and development of the human race.

"Saving the world" may sound like "motive-meddling" hogwash. It may, however, establish a fail-safe purpose for our career. Some see signs of decrease in our profession's popularity. We may blame hasty consultations, resistance to ideas that total health care is a basic right, or a public which is ill-informed. But, in fact, any "public alienation" must surely be read as a sign that we _do_ treat our job as a job and that we _do not_ constantly move ahead _of_ the thinking and needs of our patients. We have settled for "limited liability scholarship".

## ENTIRE REGIONS OF UNDERSTANDING JUST DO NOT EXIST

At the age of 14, a schoolboy in this country chooses to join one of three academic streams: classics, languages, science. Ten to fifteen years later he emerges as a specialist in his particular skill.

As ten years' participation in our profession becomes twenty or thirty, we begin to be aware that entire regions of understanding just do not exist in our map of life. Yet we give 105 good reasons to support our chosen way of living. We are in the workaholic treadmill with our travail to advance our technology. And those who talk of anything else are called "politicians". There is full scope for man's brain to enumerate sociological minutiae beyond the capability of man's mind to comprehend or understand. We produce the current situation--a world full of brilliant minds and a very shaky future. Yet in the health profession a philosophy of life, which originally moved most of us to take on the care of people, lies dormant.

Everyone would like to see the world change and be different. Everyone is waiting for someone to begin to be different. As my friend, Dr. Frank Buchman (American founder of the world work of Moral Re-Armament) used to say to us, "The best place to start is with yourself."

What is deficient in our thinking?

What is it that makes the splendid response processes of stress appear to function inadequately?

## SEVERAL CHALLENGES

At the heart of all this lie several challenges for us:

1. Do those seeking help want relief or cure?

2. Does the health service aim to relieve breakdown or to establish health?

3. Do we personally so much enjoy the techniques of analysis in our field of breakdown that we neglect the time-absorbing instruction of teaching patients the disciplines which render our intervention unnecessary?

4. Do we recognize a distinct immunology defense system in our decision-making?

5. Have we charted anchor areas in this vast sea of tides of stress-response? I have made a digest of my answer to this question in the book "Stress: an A.B.C."*

6. Do we understand the thinking of our times? If we do not, we have a limited view of our participation in the evolutionary process. What is the purpose of life, if it is not

---

*Available from Dyce, 90 Harley St., London W1N 1AF $2.00 or £1.00 in UK plus postage.

to have a role in history? And what is history if it is not about maturing of the character of the peoples on this earth?

7. How do we make the time to do creative thinking?

Today I would like to choose one only. Is there an immunology defense system within our decision-making process? From the vast range of possible aspects of this, I wish to identify three compelling overtones of ideas which influence our decisions.

## WE ARE CONFUSED BY OVERTONES OF IDEAS WE DO NOT UNDERSTAND

We will look at three items of social analysis-- three terms which carry clues to the operative power in decision-making, and to the immunology factor for our defense.

These terms are: (1.) Alienation, (2.) Dialectics, (3.) Antinomy. See them at work in British history.

## ALIENATION

By 1830 in England there ended the first phase of the Industrial Revolution. The steam engine (first invented by Watt to pump water out of coal mines) had become a tool in the beginnings of the expansion of factory design. More applications for its use jumped into existence at speed, driving spinning jennies, lathes, entire railroad systems and so forth.

Men were offered employment in the mills and factories. Their former employment in crafts, sometimes in the workshop in their own backyard, changed dramatically as they became "hands" in a factory.

The sudden loss of the need for their individual and personal creativity meant that something was lost from their lives. They were separated from, alienated from, the substance of their lives.

Previously, they had earned a livelihood by taking their very own handiwork to sell in the market place to gain the money which they personally could decide what to do with.

The vast expansion of wealth and power, and the turmoil of material advantage and disadvantage, produced the kind of economic riddles we see today.

There was a hardening of attitudes by those who were the creators of the new industries. They could support all they dreamed up for their industrial empires. There was a hardening of attitudes by those, now alienated from that part of themselves which they no longer controlled-- their individual skills.

The heart of the matter was not the juggling with the distribution of profit, nor the material benefits of the Industrial Revolution, but the effect of the expansion of knowledge on both lots of people.

The Industrial Revolution was treated as mere phenomenon. There was abication from the search for essential truth. There was willful retreat into material concerns.

Men became so involved with the manipulation of their material advantage or disadvantage they began to talk in half-truths.

It was true that there was hardship as craftsmen inevitably became "hands" in factories-- employed or unemployed as factories expanded or shrank. It was equally true the factories needed investment and leadership. That, together, was half the truth.

But what of the other half of the truth: the purpose of production, and the discovery of the inward nature of man's spirit? This was ignored and neglected. And this neglect produced the root: self-alienation from the search for the real truth about our purpose in life. Today we live in an age of half-truths. Alienation was a self-induced degenerative process.

Alienation is a word bandied about today as a cliché for a feeling of powerlessness to effect social change-- a de-personalization of the individual in a large and bureaucratic society,-- a sense of estrangement from society. This is a glib use of the word to cover up its root meaning: the lack of search for the whole truth. We, as scientists, are trained to search for the whole answer. Half-answers are no answer. Here is an area through which we can drive a team of horses---to the benefit of modern man.

There is a very fine line of division in the modern mind between the glorifying some special gift or expertise each individual possesses, and the acceptance that there is a wholly different field: the field of the spirit. We confuse the first with the second. We go up and down with success in the field of our skills, measuring our life in success or failure. We become separated from, alienated from, the over-riding field of the spirit.

## DIALECTICS

In the background of the Industrial Revolution there were thinkers and philosphers who believed that a thesis could be challenged by an antithesis and these could progress to a synthesis. A half-truth can be challenged by an antithetical half-truth so as to produce a synthesis of whole truth. The process of asking questions with a view to the discovery of synthesis is the dialectical process.

Men today, in the main, remain in a position of defending their own half-truth.

The dialectical process is rarely allowed to happen.

Men have thus erected the wrong bridge into the influencing and direction of affairs in the world. They have built computations of their own creations and assumed that the spirit in man could be satisfied by material output.

History has been off course ever since.

The dialectical process has failed to become the norm. When men meet today they pitch their negotiating position at a level, the height of which allows for a retreat to a level they were prepared to settle at in the first place: the lowest common denominator.

It takes no account of the possibilities of a discovery of a way ahead which neither had previously thought of, and which is fresh to both. So we decline into a variety of views all ending in the three letters: i-s-m-- ism: capitalism, socialism, nationalism. These are all spawned by the half-truth, materialism. Buchman asked American in 1948, "Is materialism the mother of all the 'isms'? Is materialism becoming our national ideology?"

Dialectics, then, is the positive step of accepting that the truth as I see it, my thesis, may be challenged by the truth as you see it. Both of us may make our judgement from a material point of view, backed by our facts. It must be kept quite clear that materialism is a half-truth. Our mix of well-substantiated half-truth is the thesis, which requires the antithesis of "the spirit in man" to produce the homeostatic synthesis.

ANTINOMY

We see repeatedly the goodwill of men in industry extended to the limit of yesterday's philosphy and today's dialectics: the lowest common denominator. They produce a situation of contradiction between two assertions, for each of which there seem to be adequate grounds. This is "antinomy", which is quite different from Antimony--(a brittle crystalline silvery-white metal.)

Antinomy describes the contradiction between two assertions for each of which there seem to be adequate grounds. Two logical yet apparently mutually contradictory conclusions enshrining one multi-faceted truth.

Here lies man's difficult choice in his decision-making, where two or more options appear equally right. The dilemma is constantly with us.

Antinomy supports the hardened view that each man considers that his own experience of life tells him what is right - as he sees and has experienced life. So he believes he knows what must be done. Other men hold equally clear and opposite views. Everyone is justified in saying, "My experience teaches me that 'x' is true and right." No one is justified in going on to say, "Therefore what your experience teaches you is false and wrong." That is antinomy, not synthesis. Even experience can lead to a mere half-truth. It can be a bad guide.

All that experience gives you is the growing assurance that a new dimension, as yet undiscovered, awaits revelation.

Today the world suffers from an epidemic of compromise.

At the beginnings of the universe-- after the first hot big bang-- it is calculated that there were seven elements charging around. Hydrogen and oxygen were two of these entities.

At one moment things were different from the moment before. Two atoms of hydrogen united with one of oxygen and for the very first time ever there was water.

These entities, hydrogen and oxygen, remained entities. There was no compromise. Neither gave up anything. Something new, water, produced the next stage of the evolutionary process.

This is the dimension of newness our age is faced with.

To advance in the field of electronics, the silicon chip and space technology without the equal advancement of understanding essential truth, produces alienation of an order proportionate to the difference between the horse and buggy and the space shuttle. Men lose their belief that they matter. No handout in Social Security restores the dignity of man. Human nature hardens.

There develops the idea that discussion does not work. Muscle power, fire power counts.

The view that the best that can be achieved is the lowest common denominator, leaves us with unresolved antinomy (two equal and opposite views) as the measure of success.

Human nature left in this state can readily be harnessed for materialism. Unresolved alienation and antinomy are the signs that dialectics has never been allowed to proceed to synthesis. So decision-making moves relentlessly in a materialist direction. And we fail to get the new dimension for the evolutionary process, because "human wisdom has failed".

When it is recognised that human wisdom has failed, we understand how these half-truths mobilize partisan materialism. Hitler said, "One race shall rule." Marx said, "One class shall rule."

When the whole truth is examined the spirit in man is added.

We then move from material views of the world by the addition of the antithesis of the spirit in man to a new synthesis, "One Supreme Authority shall rule."

Evolution does not depend upon us sticking with our personal experience. Evolution always goes beyond the best we know. We must allow our in-built immunology factor to produce homeostasis in our decision-making. This we do by moving through successive stages to a new dimension.

## THE NEW DIMENSION OF THE IMMUNOLOGY FACTOR

Stage One is "moral choice". Every man knows what, for him, is right. There is no question of belief, of race, of color, tied up in that element of his decision-making. It does not start at the conference table, but in the heart.

Stage Two is "obedience" to the still small voice within. It tells a person what he must do. Then he must do it.

Our own clinical work proves convincingly that you only get good at something if you are doing it every day. Then you gain wisdom. For you learn what happens. You learn, also, points of derailment where you did not really obey the rules and things went wrong. It is the same with the guidance of this inner voice--which, as a Scottish Presbyterian, I call the Voice of God.

Stage Three is "recording of proofs" that this power greater than ourselves adds a new dimension to decision-making. We begin to understand how this affects every facet of our lives.

What is the Effect of this Homeostasis in Decision-Making?

(1) Personal. The mixture of the approach to the treatment of a patient consists in presentation, skill, impact.

Presentation is all that goes into how to run the practice.

Skill is all that goes into doing the job.

Impact is all that goes into my influence on the patient.

This last is the one we have least examined.

I have learned that any time I am ill at ease with a patient there is a handicap on the success of my treatment.

Conflict during one period of my practicing career resulted in violent sick headaches. Resolution followed when I accepted that I had been in a state of conflict, trying to impress the patients in the various ways this is possible. I had a cross-current of motives, so, a cross-current in body chemistry. I was vulnerable to stress disorder.

(2) National. Incorruptible leadership is a subject which lies at the very heart of industrial method, race relations and all sorts of areas of life. It is central to the battle for power today.

I have witnessed how, by shifting my method of running my practice, men in positions of great responsibility have found people they can talk with who have no axe to grind, require no "kick-back of perks". They have common ground to rub minds about man's future, with men who have moved beyond their antinomies and alienations. I have seen men go off from our breakfast parties encouraged to do the things they know will influence the lives of nations. The success of these occasions, of course, may well lie with the fact that one's wife is fully involved with the most important role of adding much reality to the breakfast deliberations, as well as producing food. We can become so self absorbed.

CONSTELLATION AND CONSTANT INSERT INTO DECISION-MAKING

The full range of the truth brings synthesis to material values. This constellation and constant insert into our decision-making is the structure of a superior force-- a superior ideology.

I have heard one statesman patient say, "How can I, as a statesman, make a decision today which is still valid in twelve months? Science moves on so fast. No man is clever enough to calculate the expedient thing to do. Our only hope is to find and do what is right morally. Then events can never overtake us."

The stress field calls for those who will move from technical excellence (which, of course, must be basic and essential) to setting in motion the superior ideology in their world. We can have a new type of man because we, in the stress business, work so often at the cross-roads in the lives of our patients.

I find that the best time to contemplate my part in this process is early in the morning, before the telephone begins to ring.

The jargon uses of words like alienation, dialectics, antinomy, weaken and confuse our thinking. But they are some of the items which go to make the structure of a model of ideology. They indicate man's failure to face the truth about himself. It is our role to bring clarity into the situation.

That, to me, makes the study of the decision-making process the most relevant research of our time.

# THE DENTAL DISTRESS SYNDROME AND LITERATURE AVAILABILITY

A. C. Fonder, D.D.S., F.R.S.H.

Director, Medico-Dental Foundation, Inc.
Rock Falls, Illinois

The Dental Distress Syndrome (DDS) is well defined in the literature.[1-9] Distress produced by maloccluded teeth and the resultant malfunctioning musculature of the head, neck and shoulders causes spinal malposture (scoliosis, lordosis and kyphosis).[2-11] Removal of this excessive stress of dental origin allows body posture to normalize.[2-4]

Physiopathologically all systems of the body are adversely affected because DDS and Selye's GAS (General Adaptation Syndrome) are one and the same syndrome.[1-9] Widespread normalization is observed throughout all bodily systems, when the body posture normalizes.[2-18]

DDS is being treated by many specialists and professional teams including members of the American Academy of Stress and Chronic Disease, the American Academy of Craniomandibular Orthopedics, the American Academy of Physiologic Dentistry, the American Adademy for Functional Prosthodontics and select members of the International Academy of Preventive Medicine and the American Association for the Advancement of Tension Control.[13]

Obviously, when a muscle is not functioning at its physiological contracting and resting length, spasms and functional disorders will occur. So, when groups of power muscles and antagonistic holding muscles are functioning in an uncoordinated manner, physiopathologic disorders will ensue.[14] Yet the role of DDS is not well understood by general practitioners of dentistry and medicine, since it is only beginning to be taught in a few educational institutions.

The schools of osteopathy, chiropractic, physical therapy and Alexander have been quicker to recognize the role of DDS in restoration to health and in the prevention of disease. This is because they achieve results routinely through the restoration of proper posture and function.

The lack of physiologically balanced molar support that accompanies malpositioned and missing teeth and/or excessive free-way space, as observed in deep overbites, results in bruxing, muscle spasms and tempormandibular joint (TMJ) problems.[1-11]

So, the importance of all associated "dental area" muscles functioning optimally can be better understood when we consider the following:

1. Almost half of the motor and sensory function of the brain is devoted to the 'dental area'.[2-8,15]

2. The computerized brain is programmed by feedback whether it be correct or errant.[16]

3. The facial musculature instantaneously registers fear, anger, love, joy, hate, surprise and all bodily emotions.

4. Kinesiology has clearly demonstrated that each tooth is associated with a muscle and an organ of the body.[17-19]

## CONCLUSION

Since DDS plays a role in general health problems, it would seem only logical that dentistry and medicine should cooperate in research and in diagnosing and treating chronically ill patients. Medicine and dentistry should not continue to function as separate sciences.

## REFERENCES

1. A. C. Fonder, J. L. Alter, L. C. Allemand, and W. W. Monks, Malocclusion as it relates to general health, Ill. Dent. Jnl., 34:292 (1965).
2. A. C. Fonder, Spinal posture and the dental distress syndrome, essay at the annual meeting of the American Dental Association, Las Vegas (1970).
3. A. C. Fonder, The dental distress syndrome (DDS), essay at the

annual meeting of the American Dental Association, Houston (1973).
4. A. C. Fonder, Related spinal curvature and respiratory problems, essay at the annual meeting of the American Dental Association, Houston (1973).
5. A. C. Fonder, The profound effect of the 1973 Nobel prize on dentistry, Basal Facts, 2:20 (1976).
6. A. C. Fonder, Stress and the dental distress syndrome, Basal Facts, 8:119 (1976).
7. A. C. Fonder, Malocclusion, dental distress and educability, Basal Facts, 7:74 (1977).
8. A. C. Fonder, Dental stress and distress, *in* "Proceedings of the Second Annual Meeting of the American Association for the Advancement of Tension Control," F. J. McGuigan, ed., University Publications, Blacksburg, Va., (1975).
9. A. C. Fonder, "The Dental Physician," Medico-Dental Foundation, Rock Falls., Ill., (1977).
10. F. Y. A. Khoroshilkina, Y. U. M. Malygin, Y. A. A. Nesulkovsky, and V. G. Tsyplenkov, Sinusbronchial neomopathy and disturbances of posture in patients with sagittal anomalies of occulsion, Stomatologiia, 7:65 (1970).
11. H. Gelb, "Clinical Management of Head, Neck and TMJ Pain and Dysfunction," W. B. Saunders, Philadelphia-London (1977).
12. W. Barlow, "The Alexander Technique," Alfred A. Knopf, New York (1976).
13. A. C. Fonder, ed., List of academies, Basal Facts, 4:9 (1979).
14. G. B. Whatmore and D. R. Kohli, "The Physiopathology and Treatment of Functional Disorders," Grune and Stratton, Inc., New York (1974).
15. W. Penfield and T. Rasmussen, Sensory and motor hommucli, *in* "Dental Orthopaedics," The Alden Press, Oxford (1966).
16. von Holst and Mittelstaedt, Naturwissenschaften, 37:464 (1951).
17. G. Goodheart, "Applied Kinesiology," 15th edition, Goodheart Publications, Detroit (1979).
18. D. Walther, "Applied Kinesiology," Systems, D.C., Pueblo, Colo., (1976).
19. G. Eversaul, "Dental Kinesiology," Eversaul Publications, Las Vegas (1978).

## SUGGESTED ADDITIONAL READING

Enlow, D. H., 1975, "Handbook of Facial Growth," Saunders, Philadelphia- London.

Fonder, A. C., "The Physiopathology of Stressful Disorders," (to be published).

Fonder, A. C., ed., 1976-1979, Basal Facts, Doctors' Dental Service, Chicago. Vols. 1-3.

Guzay, C. M., 1979, "Biophysics of Articulation," Guzay Publications, Chicago.

Jackson, R., 1971, "The Cervical Syndrome," 3rd edition, Charles Thomas, Springfield, Ill.

Leib, M., ed., 1940-1973, Dental Concepts, American Dental Association, Chicago.

Pottinger, F. M., 1919-1959, "Symptoms of Visceral Diseases," C. V. Mosby, St. Louis.

Selye, H., 1955, "The Stress of Life," McGraw Hill, New York.

Selye, H., 1974, "Stress Without Distress," Lippincott, Philadelphia-New York.

# HYPNOTHERAPY IN THE CONTROL OF STRESS, ANXIETY AND FEAR IN DENTAL PHOBIA

G. W. Fairfull Smith, M.C., L.D.S.
Michael J. McGee, B.D.S.
Alexander M. Stewart, B.D.S.

Hypnosis Clinic
Glasgow Dental Hospital and School
Glasgow, Scotland

## INTENTION

To use hypnotherapy as a behavioral reorientation technique in the clinical dental field to aid phobics to become normal, and to teach them a method of self-regulation for controlling their stress, anxiety, and fear. To assess the value of this therapy for the next random twelve patients referred to the Hypnosis Clinic Glasgow Dental Hospital and School, Glasgow, in July of 1977.

## INTRODUCTION

Fear itself is of great value to the developing child to prevent him from injury or death. Fear is not deplorable nor abnormal as Valentine (1956) points out. Landis (1964) states that fear is a normal response to threat, real or imagined. Marks (1969) points out its usefulness since it often leads to rapid action in the face of threat, and Gray (1971) points out that it has a behavioral factor of teaching the organism. Nevertheless it is abnormal fear which generates pathological anxiety, creating stress, building up tension, and goes further in lowering the pain threshold to a point of intolerance, as has been shown by Hall and Stride (1954).

The phobiagenic factors which create dental cripples become evident when one considers Watson's (1924) model as to the origins of fear. He divides fear into two categories.

(1.) Philogenetic

(a.) Fear of pain

(b.) Fear of loss of support

(c.) Fear of a loud noise (or any extreme sensory stimulus)

(2.) Ontogenetic: Brought on by

(a.) Extraneous influences (family's and friend's experiences)

(b.) Personal experience

All or most of these factors are always present in the surgery and may all be associated with dental procedures. The authors suggest that this is the reason for the universal fear of dental treatment. Robbins (1962) and Levitt (1968) report that out of a large sample group of people 2% were minimally anxious about their teeth, yet 89% were specifically fearful of dental treatment. This fear is unrelated to education, age, sex, racial, religious and ethnic differences. They also report that in the fear factor of general illness only the fear of cancer is greater than the fear of dental treatment.

Janis (1958) found that fear of treatment of dental cavities is greater than the fear of minor or major surgery. Extreme dental phobia appears to be in the category of 6% to 16% of any population as several studies have shown. (Gale and Ayer, 1969; Marks, 1969, Kleinknecht et al., 1973, and Kegeles, 1963). Gall (1965) states that a further 40 to 50% of the population is dental phobic to a lesser degree. In this the milder form, dental phobic illness prevents optimum attendance and full co-operation of the patient during treatment, only attending for treatment when there is severe pain associated with their teeth. In the more severe forms, 16%, the patient totally avoids dental care (Gerscham et al., 1976).

## Hypnosis

That there is a group of biological behavioral phenomena which collectively has been classified as hypnosis is an accepted fact (British Medical Journal, 1955). Barry Wyke, (1977) professor of neurophysiology at the Royal College of Surgeons, London, England, says that as yet it is impossible to define hypnosis in phenomenological terms due to the lack of hard data on the intimate specific workings of the brain cells, so an operant definition must suffice.

This is the result of empirical observations and the computer analysis of thousands of results of implanted micro-electrodes in the brains of animals and humans. This biological behavioral phenomenon may be defined as an altered perceptual status of whatever duration. Its characteristic difference from any other altered perceptual states depends on the involvement of the mechanisms of attention, and habituation. These two mechanisms are the sine qua non of hypnosis. This phenomenon appears to be modulated by a bundle of nerve cells in the mid-brain called the reticular formation when it functions in conjunction with the limbic system, the long-term memory cells, and the reticulofrontal projection system.

## DISCUSSION

The twelve dental phobics surveyed were a random choice of the next twelve consecutive referrals to the Hypnosis Clinic. There were four males and eight females of ages ranging from 8 to 37 years old, with the average age being 19 years. They all had extreme fear of dental treatment. The eight year-old patient had not been to a dentist for four years and that was the shortest period of avoidance. The longest was 27 years. Three patients reported fainting when they had gone to dental surgeries to make appointments. They all had other neuroses in conjunction with their dental phobic disease. The dental phobia is often only one symptom of many, signifying that all is not well.

The patients reported the following symptoms:

| | |
|---|---|
| Claustrophobia (1) | Pathological quick temper (1) |
| Plane phobias (2) | Excessive blushing (2) |
| Agoraphobias (3) | Excessive perspiration (1) |
| Depression (3) | Excessive anxiety (12) |
| Obesity problem (1) | Bruxism (3) |
| Nail biters (4) | Insomnia (1) |

Nine of the twelve intimated to being on regular psychotropic drugs, the other three from time to time.

Willoughby's personality schedule (Wilkinson and Latif, 1974) was used to assess normality/neuroticism changes. Due to the very short time taken from the first to the last session of treatment, there were no significant changes in the readings, but they were noted for future assessment.

A phobia profile was obtained by devising a very simple self evaluation phobia heirarchy-index schedule. This proved to be very useful as an indication for the forming of specific therapeutic suggestions for the desensitization. It was also a very accurate and useful subjective measurement of the degree of betterment. A copy of this schedule is attached (see appendix A).

The best improvement of the phobia profile was from 14 to 43 signifying a 307% improvement. The average improvement was 217%. The patients were given one-half hour sessions at weekly intervals. The most number of visits was eight, and the least two. The average number of visits was 4.67.

The Stanford Hypnotic Clinical Scale was taken at the commencement of treatment. There was one non-hypnotizable and one scored 100%; the average score was 55%. (Hilgard and Hilgard, 1975-a).

METHODS

The patients were all induced by the Glasgow Dental Hospital method (F. Smith 1976-a) then they were taught a system of self-relaxation in the waking state. The one chosen for its simplicity was a modification of Stein's "Clenched Fist" technique (Stein 1965).

They were then taught self-hypnotherapy, (R. Smith, 1970). It is imperative to teach the patient self-confidence and independence, an ability to self-regulate himself phychophysiologically, and also to continue his own therapy and treatment at home. They were requested to do this daily at home at least once, if possible three sessions of five minutes to 10 minutes.

Four distinct psychotherapies were built into the self-hypnotherapy.

(1.) A deep relaxation method (Jacobson, 1938) was taught. This triggers off the trophotropic cells around the hypothalumus creating biological recuperative mechanisms producing calmness, reducing stress, sublimating tension, anxiety and fear---mechanisms described by Hess (1924), electrically triggered by Delgado et al., (1954), and called the "Relaxation Response" by Benson et al., 1975).

(2.) A reality therapy was given to boost the patient's ego, and thus hep him control his inadequacy and insufficiency and help the integration and maturation of his personality (Hartland, 1965, Stanton, 1975, F. Smith, 1976-b).

(3.) Wolpe's (1969) "Reciprocal Inhibition" therapy of desensitization, or Stample and Levis's "Implosion" technique (1966) was interwoven into the self-hypnotherapy to help the patient overcome fear and anxiety. The patient forms new attitudes towards dental treatment.

(4.) The patient was taught "glove anaesthesia" (Hilgard and Hilgard 1975-b) as a modulator of pain for surgical procedures. The extent of pain control obtained is very subjective and varies from dermal-analgesia to deep anaesthesia. Nevertheless it often is enough to be useful in conjunction with local anaesthesia.

## RESULTS

Ten patients accepted dental treatment normally after their course of hypnotherapy, without any stress, anxiety, or fear. One of these patients managed to control surgical pain completely and had all his subsequent treatments without any form of pharmacological help. The other nine patients accepted their dental treatment in conjunction with local anaesthesia, relative analgesia or general anaesthesia.

Five went back to their family general dental practitioners and five had their treatment carried out by student operators in the hospital.

One ten-year-old girl had a reasonable depth of hypnosis but still refused local anesthesia. She was counted as a failure even through she subsequently had her treatment with general anesthesia. One boy did not complete his hypnotherapy course. He was the non-hypnotizable. All the concommitant neuroses were also resolved with no specific suggestions given for them. They also reported that they had cut down their psychotropic drugs immediately, and after two years they were all free from the need to take them regularly.

## CONCLUSION

Hypnosis appears to be an effective self-regulation aid and with other therapies able to re-orientate attitudes, boost ego, control stress, anxiety, fear and a degree of pain. Like all other therapies it has its limitations, but 83% success rate in a random group of people is reasonably good. Especially so, as these ten patients on a follow-up assessment after two years were still attending routine dental treatment without any stress or fear. As other neuroses were also spontaneously influenced it would appear that the hypnotherapy per se regardless of depth helped the patients to integrate their personalities.

ACKNOWLEDGEMENT

We wish to acknowledge the constant encouragement, help and support given to us by Dean James Ireland, Director of Dental Studies, Glasgow University; Professor Michael R. Bond, Psychological Medicine, Glasgow University; Mr. Andrew Carmichael, head of the Department of Conservation, Glasgow Dental Hospital and School; Mr. James Gall the Deputy-Chief Dental Officer, Scottish Home and Health Deparment, the staff of the Glasgow Dental Hospital and School, and the Greater Glasgow Health Board.

## APPENDIX A

### THE GLASGOW DENTAL HOSPITAL - DENTAL PHOBIA INDEX

#### INSTRUCTIONS

The questions in this schedule are intended to indicate various phobic traits. It is not a test in any sense because there are no right and wrong answers to any of the questions in this schedule.

After each question you will find a row of numbers whose meaning is given below. All you have to do is to draw a ring around the number that describes you best.

0. means "no", "never", "not at all" etc.
1. means "somewhat", "sometimes", "A little" etc.
2. means "about as often as not", "an average amount" etc.
3. means "usually", "a good deal", "rather often" etc.
4. means "practically always", "entirely", "yes" ect.

| | | | | | | |
|---|---|---|---|---|---|---|
| 1. | Do you brush your teeth daily? | 0 | 1 | 2 | 3 | 4 |
| 2. | Do you visit your dentist every six months? | 0 | 1 | 2 | 3 | 4 |
| 3. | Do you select your own toothpaste? | 0 | 1 | 2 | 3 | 4 |
| 4. | Do you choose your own toothbrush? | 0 | 1 | 2 | 3 | 4 |
| 5. | Do you like the smell of the dental surgery? | 0 | 1 | 2 | 3 | 4 |
| 6. | Do you like the smell of the drilling? | 0 | 1 | 2 | 3 | 4 |
| 7. | Do you tolerate injections? | 0 | 1 | 2 | 3 | 4 |
| 8. | Can you stand the sight of blood? | 0 | 1 | 2 | 3 | 4 |
| 9. | Do you like a dental general anaesthetic? | 0 | 1 | 2 | 3 | 4 |

10. Can you stand the noise of drilling? 0 1 2 3 4

11. Can you tolerate the noise of extractions? 0 1 2 3 4

12. Do you feel normally composed the week you are going to the dentist? 0 1 2 3 4

13. Do you feel normal the day before you go to the dentist? 0 1 2 3 4

14. Do you feel normal the day you are going to the dentist? 0 1 2 3 4

15. Do you feel composed when you ring the dentist's door bell? 0 1 2 3 4

16. Do you feel composed when you go into the waiting room? 0 1 2 3 4

17. Do you feel calm and composed when you sit in the waiting room? 0 1 2 3 4

18. Do you feel composed when your name is called out? 0 1 2 3 4

19. Do you know your dentist's name? 0 1 2 3 4

20. Do you feel the dentist is friendly? 0 1 2 3 4

REFERENCES

Benson, H., and Klipper, M. Z., 1975, "The Relaxation Response," Collins, London.

*British Medical Journal*, 1955, Medical use of hypnotism, Supplementary Report of B.M.A. Council, App. X, 190.

Delgado, M. M. R., Roberts, W. W., and Miller, N. E., 1954, Learning motivated by electrical stimulation of the brain, *Am. Jnl. Physiol.*, 179:587.

Fairfull Smith, G. W., (a), 1976, The modulation of fear anxiety and pain with hypnosis, *SAAD Dig.*, 3:76.

Fairfull Smith, G. W., (b), 1976, A therapy for smokers, *Proc. Brit. Soc. Med. Dent. Hyp.*, 2:46.

Gale, E. N., and Ayer, W. A., 1969, Treatment of dental phobias, *Jnl. Amer. Dental Assoc.*, 78:130.

Gall, J., 1965, Deputy Chief Dental Officer, Scottish Home and Health Department, Personal communication.

Gercham, J. A., Burrows, G. D., and Reade, P. C., 1976, The role of hypnosis in dental phobic illness, Australian Jnl. of Clin. Hyp., 4:58.

Gray, J., 1971, "The Psychology of Fear and Stress," World University Library, Weidenfield and Nicolson, London.

Hall, K. R. L., and Stride, E., 1954, The varying response to pain in psychiatric disorder, Brit. Jnl. Med. Psy., 27:28.

Hartland, J., 1965, "Medical and Dental Hypnosis," Bailliere, Tindall, and Cassell, London.

Hess, W. R., 1924, "Das Zwischenhirn: Syndrome, Lokalizationen, Funktionen," 2nd ed., Schwabe, Basel.

Hilgard, E., and Hilgard, J., 1975, "Hypnosis in the Relief of Pain," Kaufman, New York.

Jacobson, E., 1938, "Progressive Relaxation," University of Chicago Press, Chicago.

Janis, I. L., 1958, "Psychological Stress," Wiley, New York.

Kegeles, S. S., 1963, Some motives for seeking preventive dental treatment, Jnl. Am. Dent. Assoc., 7:90.

Kleinknecht, R. A., Klepac, R. K., and Alexander, L. D., 1973, Origins and characteristics of fear of dentistry, Jnl. of Am. Dent. Assoc., 86:842.

Landis, C., "Varieties of Psychopathological Experience," F. A. Mettler, ed., Holt, Reinhart, and Winston, New York.

Levitt, E. E., 1968, "Psychology of Anxiety," Paladin Granada, London.

Marks, I., 1969, "Fears and Phobias," Heineman Medical, London.

Robbins, P. R., 1962, Some explorations into the nature of anxieties relating to illness, Genet. Psy. Mono., 66:91.

Roy Smith, S., 1970, The significance of autohypnosis in dentistry, Br. Jnl. Clin. Hyp., 12:8.

Stample, T. G., and Levis, D. G., "Handbook of Direct Behavior Psychotherapies," University of North Carolina Press, Chapel Hill.

Stanton, H., 1975, Ego-enhancement through positive suggestions, Australian Jnl. of Clin. Hyp., 3:32.

Stein, C., 1965, The clenched fist as a hypnotic procedure in clinical psychotherapy, Am. Jnl. Clin. Hyp., 6:113.

Valentine, C. W., 1975, "The Normal Child," Pelican Books, England.

Watson, J. B., 1924, "Behaviorism," Norton, New York.

Wolpe, J., 1958, "Psychotherapy by Reciprocal Inhibition," Standford University Press, Stanford, Calif.

Wyke, B. S., 1977, Hypnosis as a neurological phenomenon, Symposium at Royal Society of Medicine, London.

# TENSION AND HEADACHES

# GROUP RELAXATION IN THE TREATMENT OF MIGRAINE

## A MULTIFACTORIAL APPROACH

Jane Madders, Dip. Phys. Ed., M.C.S.P.

Physiotherapist, Author, Broadcaster
Birmingham, England

## INTRODUCTION

Migraine is a disorder of blood vessels and was described over 5,000 years ago. Its essential feature is vascular instability, especially of the arteries, arterioles and microcirculation of the head and neck (Wolff 1963). The causes, symptoms and trigger factors are varied, and the treatment described is also multifactorial. It is an attempt to treat the whole person in his environmental setting and to provide a self-help method which does not depend upon drugs.

Migraine has been defined as recurrent headaches, widely varied in intensity, frequency and duration, usually unilateral at onset and often associated with nausea and vomiting. It is familial, and there is freedom from symptoms between attacks. In some cases the headache is preceded by or associated with sensory, motor and mood changes and these may be alarming to the individual who is unaware of the cause. The changes include visual phenomena of shimmering lights, zigzags, blank spots and distortion of shapes. Though to the sufferer these may seem to last for hours, they usually last about twenty minutes. There may be motor disturbances with lurching gait and some individuals experience embarrassing speech difficulties and tingling or numbness of fingers. Sustained contraction of the muscles of the neck and scalp augment the pain, and pain itself raises levels of arousal.

Migraine causes much distress, absence from work and disruption of family life with consequent feelings of guilt at letting people down without warning. There is still much to be discovered about the basic cause, but a pattern is beginning to emerge. There is an inherent disposition towards migraine, sensitivity to external stimuli such as bright lights, loud noises, smells, and vivid patterns.

There is much controversy as to whether there is such a thing as a "migraine personality," and sufferers will be relieved to learn that the myth of neuroticism and hypochondriasis has been demolished (Philips 1975). There is some evidence of characteristics shared by migraineurs. Many score highly in guilt-proneness in that they feel guilty if high standards are not met or if work cannot be completed to time. Allied to this is a tendency to react to criticism with bodily responses more suitable for a physical threat. My own experience with hundreds of migraine patients bears this out and has modified my methods of teaching--so that small stages of success are noted and shortcomings ignored.

Thus the gun is loaded, but it requires a trigger to spark off an attack. At one time there seemed to be little in common among the wide and often bizarre range of trigger factors. These include dietary ones such as chocolate, cheese, citrus fruits, red wine and fasting; change in any form, whether an alteration in hormone levels, changes in weather, holidays, travel. Fatigue and high levels of arousal are probably the most common precipitants, whether the agent is pleasant or unpleasant, and include anger, excitement, anxiety and even sheer joy if the reaction is intense and prolonged. The research of Hanington (1973) and her team has shown that all these factors are concerned with vaso-active amines. The dietary factors include these: tyramine, histamine, and phenylethylamine. Stress elicits the output of catecholamines. It appears that migraine sufferers lack the wherewithal to render therse amines harmless.

I have given this overall picture to show where group relaxation plays a part in the treatment of migraine. It can provide techniques for lowering levels of arousal, give information about the nature of migraine and by partner-assisted teaching and group discussions contribute towards mutual understanding and support.

## METHOD

In order to assess the efficacy of group methods, a training course was held for physiotherapists, health visitors and teachers with special qualifications in health education. This was done to eliminate the effects of a single personality upon results. The teachers then conducted a series of seven weekly classes with 12-20 men and women, all of whom had been diagnosed as having migraine, some very severely. They were referred either by their general practitioners or by the Birmingham Migraine Clinic. Classes lasted 90 minutes and were held in the afternoon at the clinic or in the evenings in a variety of halls and homes. Inevitably there was self-selection because only those who were aware that stress was a major factor in precipitating their migraine were strongly motivated to give up much free time to attend classes. A total of 149 patients attended at least five of the sessions

At the introductory session a talk was given about migraine, stress and relaxation. Simple biofeedback apparatus (GSR with an audible signal) was used to illustrate the bodily effects of general arousal, whether caused by the fear response to a noise or in answering a question or recalling an embarrassing event. It also demonstrated the possibility of exerting some voluntary control over autonomic function. The apparatus was later used at one of the group discussions but it only augmented teaching and in no way replaced relaxation training.

Every session included muscle relaxation and a special feature was the use of partners to assess progress and to help them become aware of the difference in quality of muscle tension and relaxation. By changing partners each week patients became aware of the wide range of individual differences in the ability to relax and they all were involved in the teaching process. There was an added bonus in that the friendly physical contact was a factor in releasing tension.

Massage of shoulders and forehead by partners was introduced in the second and subsequent sessions. Physiologically, massage stimulates the flow of blood, helps reduce muscle tension and its associated pain. It does more than this, however, for there is a subtle calming down of the whole body, a reduction of anxiety and the receiver is enabled to feel rather than to think. In many cultures touching is discouraged, the slightest brushing against another requires an instant apology, and people go to great lengths to avoid touching each other. Massage of the objective kind used in the classes for forehead and shoulders, over clothes if necessary, is acceptable and manifestly enjoyed. However, the point is made that the resultant relaxation must be recognized so that it can be reproduced later without the aid of a partner.

A brief spell of relaxation sitting upright in an office type chair emphasizes the need to snatch short periods of relaxation in any situation when the pressures are mounting. Full, general relaxation followed, lying on the floor with bright lights dimmed. After fifteen minutes or more, patients were roused and light refreshments served (fasting can precipitate a migraine in some sensitive subjects) as they sat in small discussion groups of not more than six in each. The discussions were structured and nonthreatening so that every member could talk freely with no acknowledged expert present on whom to rely.

The earlier discussions were concerned with migraine, each member telling the others about the characteristics of the attacks and the various trigger factors. Later the emphasis changed to more positive aspects of relaxation introduced to daily living situations, sharing successes and problems. The emphasis was on sharing information and giving mutual support. At the end of each session the class reassembled and questions were put to the teacher who gave suggestions for the week's practice at home. At the final class, husbands, wives or close friends were invited to attend to learn more about migraine and how best to support relaxation practice. Some patients chose to attend another series, others practised on their own.

More recently, patients have been shown how to monitor the pain trigger areas in forehead, scalp and neck. These have been described by Dr. Hay, consultant at the Birmingham Migraine Clinic (1979) and he has shown that some patients can be trained to become aware of the increase in tenderness of these areas shortly before an attack. In this way relaxation practice can be increased, and daily living situations modified so that levels of arousal can be lowered.

## RESULTS

A postal questionnaire was sent to 149 participants three to twelve months after classes had ended. Some 130 replies were received.

79% reported that since attending the classes they considered they were "better."

20% reported that their condition was "the same."

One woman was "worse."

73% reported that they were either taking no drugs or fewer than before.

These results are largely similar to those in a previous pilot study (Hay and Madders, 1971) when more sophisticated and complex questionnaires were used to assess degrees of intensity, frequency and duration of attacks.

## DISCUSSION

Relaxation is not a "cure" for migraine, but it can provide a valuable self-help method to raise the threshold to attacks, enabling many patients to alleviate them and in some cases to eliminate them, and lessening the use of drugs. There are undoubtedly flaws in the design of the experiment: there has been no overall follow-up after the first year, and the multifactorial nature of the classes make for difficulties. However, the results obtained over several years point to the value of group methods of relaxation, using biofeedback, partner assistance, massage and group dicsussions to augment the teaching. It has been directly applied to daily living situations. It appears to be most successful among those who are well motivated and who recognize stress and fatigue as major factors precipitating their attacks. It is least successful among those depending upon frequent doses of ergotomine tartrate drugs when their headaches may be the result of over use (Wilkinson 1976).

## REFERENCES

Hanington, E., 1973, "Migraine," Priory Press, London.
Hay, K. M., 1979, Pain thresholds in migraine, The Practit., 222:827.
Hay, K. M., and Madders, J., 1971, Migraine treated by relaxation, Jnl. Royal Col. Gen. Practit., 21:664.
Madders, J., 1979, "Stress and Relaxation," Martin Dunitz, Ltd., London.
Philips, C., 1975, "Psychology and Medicine," Temple Smith, London.
Wilkinson, M., Feb. 1976, Ergotomine tartrate overdose, Brit. Med. Jnl., 525.

# SELF-CONTROL OF TENSION HEADACHE

Kenneth A. Holroyd, Ph.D.

Professor of Psychology
Ohio University
Athens, Ohio

Frank Andrasik, Ph.D.

Professor of Psychology
State University of New York
Albany, New York

I would like to briefly review some of our research on the treatment of chronic tension headache. I am particularly interested in reactions from people who are as sophisticated in the use of relaxation as this group, because our findings suggest that the learned control of muscle tension may play a less important role in the self-control of tension headache than we had previously thought.

The exact etiology of tension headache remains unclear. However there is a general consensus that tension headache (1.) is an individual response to psychological stress and (2.) may result from the sustained contraction of skeletal muscles about the face, scalp, neck, and shoulders.

Behavioral approaches to tension headache have focused on the muscle tension that is assumed to contribute to tension headache. Generally it has been found that both relaxation training and EMG biofeedback are effective in helping many tension headache sufferers control their headaches. However, the headache sufferer's ability to control EMG activity following treatment is typically observed to be unrelated to, or at best, weakly related to headache improvement. This is, of course, puzzling if you assume these procedures are effective because they teach clients to control muscle tension.

The situation becomes even more complex if you ask clients following treatment what they are doing differently in situations that previously elicited tension headache. At least what we have found is that following biofeedback our clients report a wide variety of changes in the way they cope, cognitively and behaviorally, with stressful situations. They may report more assertive behavior, the avoidance of stressful situations, the rational reevaluation of headache related stresses when these factors have never been mentioned during treatment.

Since our clients seemed to be telling us that they were controlling their headaches by altering the way they coped with headache-eliciting situations, we decided to see what would happen if we dispensed with the biofeedback altogether and, instead, taught headache sufferers to cope more effectively with daily life stresses.

Drawing upon the work of cognitive-behavior therapists (e.g., Arron Beck, Donald Meichenbaum and Marvin Goldfried) we designed a brief therapeutic program that focused changing the ways clients coped with headache-related stresses. We focused on identifying: (1.) the cues that triggered tension and anxiety; (2.) how the client respond when under stress; (3.) and the client's thoughts prior to becoming aware of tension, while tense and subsequently; and (4.) the way in which these cognitions contribute to the client's tension and headache. Relationships between situational variables (ex. criticism from spouse), client's thoughts (ex. "I can't do anything right") and emotional response and symptom (ex. depression and headache) were elucidated. As soon as clients became fluent at verbalizing cognitions associated with distress they were instructed to deliberately interrupt the sequence of covert events preceding their emotional response at the earliest possible moment. In order to do this clients employed signs of impending distress as a signal to engage in cognitive strategies incompatible with the further occurrance of cognitive stress responses. The strategies provided were designed to enable clients to employ each of three main types of intrapsychic coping responses that have been identified by Lazarus and his co-workers: cognitive reappraisal, attention deployment and fantasy.

We began by comparing this stress-coping training with frontal biofeedback (Holroyd, Andrasik & Westbrook, 1977) when both treatments were accompanied by counter-demand instructions. We randomly assigned 31 chronic tension headache sufferers to either stress-coping training, biofeedback or a wait-list control group. We found stress-coping therapy to be highly effective in reducing tension headaches (77% improvement in headache symptoms at 6 week follow-up). In fact in a recent follow-up study we found these improvements were maintained two years later. We have also

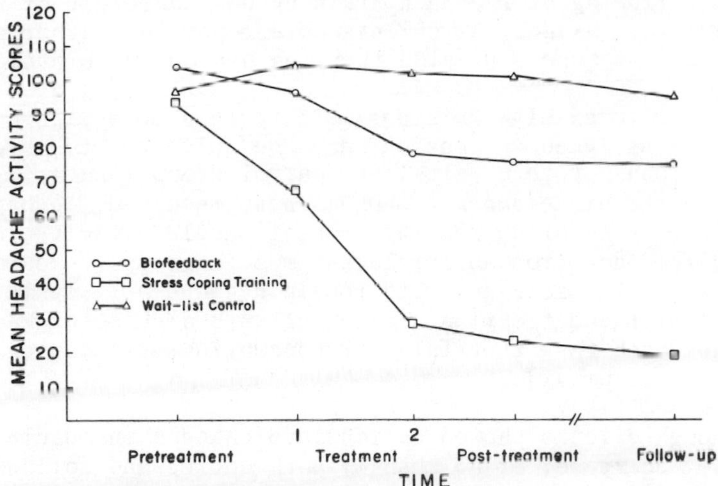


Fig. 1. Figure shows differences in mean headache activity between those using stress-coping training, biofeedback, and the wait-list control group. Copyright by Plenum Publishing Corp., 1977, Holroyd, K., Andrasik, F., and Westbrook, T. "Cognitive Control of Tension Headache." Cognitive Theraphy and Research. 1977. Vol. 1, 128. Reprinted by permission.

replicated these findings in a second study (Holroyd and Andrasik, 1978) as have other investigators (Kremsdorf, 1978). Thus we are reasonably confident that a cognitive-behavioral approach to tension headache is a viable one. Results from our second study, however, suggested that if we taught clients to monitor their responses to stress so they were able to recognize the insidious onset of headache symptoms, they would change the ways they were coping with these stressful situations even when we didn't teach any coping skills. This suggests it may be less crucial to provide clients with specific coping responses than to insure they monitor the insidious onset of symptoms and are capable of engaging in some sort of cognitive or behavioral response incompatible with the further exacerbation of symptoms. This response need not be relaxation and in certain situations where relaxation is inappropriate probably should not be relaxation.

This brings us back to the question of what accounts for the effectiveness of biofeedback. In our first study (Holroyd et al., 1977) clients who received stress-coping training reduced their headache symptoms without knowing self-control of EMG activity, while most clients who learned self-control of EMG activity through biofeedback training failed to show headache improvement. Thus there was no relationship between the learned control of EMG activity and headache improvement. We began to wonder whether the headache improvements we observed following biofeedback training were a result of the cognitive and behavioral changes our clients were reporting rather than from the self-control of muscle tension they learned during biofeedback.

In order to examine this possibility in a more rigorous fashion we randomly assigned 40 tension headache sufferers to three biofeedback groups or to a wait-list control group (Andrasik and Holroyd, 1979). In the biofeedback groups clients received feedback for either increasing or decreasing frontal muscle activity, or they received feedback from an irrelevant muscle group (forearm flexor), so that frontal muscle activity remained constant. It is important to note that these treatments allow clients a sense of mastery over the biofeedback task that false or noncontingent feedback control groups fail to provide.

Although clients showed appropriate changes in muscle tension (increase, decrease, or no change) both during and following treatment, all clients were led to believe they were learning to reduce tension levels. Clients in all three treatment groups showed substantial reductions in headache activity relative to a wait-list control group, irrespective of the actual feedback they received. Thus the learned reduction of EMG activity appeared to play a minor role in the outcomes that were obtained with biofeedback. Interview data further suggested that clients in all the treatment groups controlled their headaches by changing the way they coped with headache eliciting situations.

Other results from our laboratory (Holroyd, Andrasik & Noble, in press) suggest that the outcomes obtained without biofeedback cannot be dismissed as resulting simply from exposure to a credititible treatment. Thus exposure to a highly credible treatment does not necessarily result in symptom improvement when clients are discouraged from changing the ways they cope with headache eliciting situations.

## CONCLUSION

Those of us who are interested in biofeedback or relaxation training have been too ready to attribute the therapeutic gains we observe to the learned control of physiological activity that we so painstakingly teach during treatment. So ready are we to make this attribution that we seldom measure any other variables. Often we even fail to ask our clients exactly what they are doing differently in symptom eliciting situations when they show improvement. I would like to suggest that we are not likely to understand the therapeutic effects of biofeedback or relaxation training unless we pay more attention to the ways our clients are actually coping with the stresses they are confronting in their lives.

There is a considerable body of evidence (see Holroyd, 1979) which suggests that the way we cope with stress can influence our health. However, there is no particular coping response that is appropriate in all contexts. Muscle relaxation may often be helpful. In other instances assertive behavior, withdrawal, rational re-evaluation of environmental demands or other coping activities may be more appropriate. Therefore, treatments that ignore the demands of particular headache-eliciting situations, and provide clients with only one coping response (e.g. muscle relaxation), may prove less effective than treatments that provide clients with a more flexible set of coping skills.

## REFERENCES

Andrasik, E., and Holroyd, K., 1979, A test of the specific effects of the biofeedback treatment of tension headache, Submitted for publication.

Holroyd, K., 1979, Stress, coping and the treatment of stress-related illness, in "Behavioral Approaches in Medicine: Application and Analysis," J. R. McNamara, ed., Plenum, New York.

Holroyd, K., and Andrasik, F., 1978, Coping and the self-control of chronic tension headache, Jnl. of Consult. and Clin. Psych., 46:1036.

Holroyd, K., Andrasik, F., and Noble, J., in press, A comparison of EMG biofeedback and a credible pseudotherapy in treating tension headache, Jnl. of Behav. Med.

Holroyd, K., Andrasik, F., and Westbrook, T., 1977, Cognitive control of tension headache, Cogn. Therapy and Res., 1:121.

Kremsdorf, R. B., 1978, Biofeedback and cognitive skills training: An evaluation of their relative efficacy, Paper presented at the Biofeedback Society of America, Albuquerque.

# TENSION AND PSYCHIATRY

# PREVENTIVE PSYCHIATRY

W. Horsley Gantt, M.D.

President, AAATC
Director, Pavlovian Laboratory (Retired)
John Hopkins Medical School
Baltimore, Maryland

ABSTRACT*

Prevention means the elimination of the disease, not the early detection and treatment in the early stages. Logically the prevention of psychiatric disease depends upon the discovery of the cause. Much work is being done on the causes of neuroses and psychoses, and some have been discovered. However, there is no proven cause of the main psychosis, schizophrenia. But a limited advance is possible before we know the exact cause or causes.

What I propose before we know the complete and specific cause or causes is (1.) to make use of the knowledge we have, and (2.) a systematic study to determine if not the cause, the basis for susceptibility for the development of neurotic breakdown, so that the prevention can be instituted before the disease actually appears. This means that we would know which individuals have a predisposition to become psychotic and that measures could be taken to prevent the actual breakdown.

There are already studies that indicate we have a reasonable method of detecting susceptibility in both dogs and humans. The laboratory test for dogs is as follows:

After establishing positive and negative conditional reflexes in a dog, a slight amount of stress is produced by increasing the difficulty of differentiation by bringing the conditional stimuli

*Abstract only available.

closer together. The effect on the behavior of the dog is measured by secretion, cardiovascular and respiratory responses, metabolic changes, motor behavior, and duration of these disturbances.

A somewhat different procedure has been used with human patients. A study in the psychiatric clinic uses the method of the conditional reflex, viz., introducing a slight stress using discrimination, and measuring (1.) the extent of the disturbance in motor activity, cardiovascular and respiratory functions and (2.) the deviation of the disturbances.

We have shown that the psychiatric patient reveals marked differences from the normal individual. A number of other studies--genetics, biochemistry, etc.--indicate susceptibility. A logical study would have the examination of numbers of children of school age by appropriate tests and follow them for a decade to verify the laboratory and clinical studies, such as is done with incipient cardiac cases.

This could enable us not only to counsel and protect the susceptible individual but to develop special drugs and appropriate methods for prevention. Thus, we would not wait for the early symptoms but act on the basis of susceptibility to breakdown.

# A HAPPY CONCLUSION OF A PSYCHOANALYTICAL PSYCHOTHERAPY BY PROGRESSIVE RELAXATION AND SYSTEMATIC DESENSITIZATION

Yves Chesni, M.D.

Neuropsychiatrist
Geneva, Switzerland

A few years ago, passing through Heathrow Airport, I was surprised to see a huge notice which said: TIME IS MONEY. This is only partly true: time is a field of our development which is not only a matter of economics.

In this way, therapeutically speaking, we have the duty to treat our patients as quickly and as economically as possible but also as well as possible, which may demand time and money, first of all for the training of highly qualified therapists.

We know the long duration of psychoanalytical treatments. Freud was the first to insist on the "never ending psychoanalysis." He pointed out the importance of reinforcing the ego, which must become able to dominate, in an appropriate way, both instincts and stress (which depends on internal and external conditions) yet he didn't know any means of doing so except deep psychoanalysis.

Our "psychoanalytically-oriented psychotherapies" are often shorter but not always more successful, although we don't refuse the occasional help of pharmacological means, as long as they don't mask the symptons too much, as these are the cornerstone of the psychoanalytical treatment.

Jacobson's progressive relaxation may also require months and years. But contrary to the psychoanalysis, which needs the therapeutical relationship until the end, progressive relaxation can be taught and learned relatively quickly and the following long practice, which is required for the "automatization", for the creation of new habits, can be continued alone without the help of the therapist. Under these conditions, relatively quick and inexpensive group-training can be provided, as Professor McGuigan showed us recently.

Although (or perhaps because) this is a synthetic method, Wolpe's systemetic desensitization may be shorter, particularly when it is based on a relatively hasty relaxation and on a quick grouping of anxiety-making situations.

I will now suggest that certain forms of synthesis between psychoanalysis, relaxation and desensitization may sometimes be possible, useful and relatively brief.

## THE ENDING OF A PSYCHOANALYTICAL PSYCHOTHERAPY BY PROGRESSIVE RELAXATION AND SYSTEMATIC DESENSITIZATION

I practiced psychoanalysis for a long time before practicing relaxation and desensitization. I first applied relaxation and desensitization with patients during psychoanalysis, because of the tendency of the pure psychoanalytical treatment to be unending or for other reasons. The following case belongs to the first category.

For four or five years I psychoanalyzed a man of about 40, married, having received at birth both a strong constitution and terrible parents. From this combination and from various other circumstances resulted enormous affective troubles contrasting with a high professional formation and great social responsibilities. Among these troubles it was possible to observe persisting strong oral, anal and genital sadistic tendencies, with a previously conscious, later unconscious fantasy related to an infantile conception of intercourse: during intercourse the penis of the man penetrates and bursts the penis of the woman and thereby sadistically castrates her; from the bloody remains the child will be born. He was frightened at the idea of being castrated when he looked at naked women. He had feared for a long time that his wife's vagina was a guillotine-trap.

As he did as a child with his mother (and at this time perhaps partly justified) he continued as an adult to slice social partners who were sometimes either aggressed by him or aggressing him, and sometimes exaggeratedly idealized. At the same time he loved and admired me, and wanted to be loved and admired by me, he hated me. His first transference dream was terrific: I was introducing a pneumatic-drill into his anus. A few weeks later, he dreamt he was breaking the head of God and from time to time he wanted to do the same with me during the sessions. Another fear was of being abandoned and perhaps that had sometimes been one of the secret desires of his mother.

The results of the psychoanalysis were remarkable. The insight improved greatly and the most obvious symptoms disappeared. However, a sort of stagnation finally appeared, with the risk of a never ending treatment.

Without going into details I shall just say that, in this case, a progressive relaxation and a systematic desensitization seem to have provided a quick and good termination of the treatment. The persisting remains of repression, resistance and transference, the secondary benefits of the neurosis, certain almost bodily habits -- all factors of which inertia could cause an indefinite prolongation of a pure psychoanalytical treatment--were quickly eliminated. However it is still too soon to evaluate the long term results.

## ABOUT PSYCHOANALYSIS AND SYSTEMATIC DESENSITIZATION: A "STRUCTURELIST" HYPOTHESIS CONCERNING THE MECHANISM OF HEALING BY SYSTEMATIC DESENSITIZATION

It is known that deep relaxation can provide us with spiritual peace and improve our insight about ourselves as well as our understanding of the whole of reality. I shall only concentrate on the systematic desensitization.

Behavior therapy (which has become as introspective as behavioral and which will probably also finally take into account the Freudian unconsciousness) considers that the treatment of the present and conscious symptoms (seen or unseen from the outside) is equal to the treatment of the entire illness. As psychoanalysis does with the analysis of the transference and the normalization of the human relationship, systematic desensitization considers the present time. Contrary to the psychoanalysis it doesn't tend to remember or reconstruct the past. How does it heal old, partly unconscious, pathological processes?

The psychoanalyst is used to thinking in a "structuralist" way. He takes into account the general phenomenona of displacement, substitution and symbolization. So he tends to think that the generalization of beneficial effects of systematic desensitization come from the putting out or from the normalization of common pathological structures. With these, all past, present and future situations which contain them (as well as differences), all possible substitution symptoms are treated or prevented at the same time.

Yet, according to Wolpe, a large number of failures of systematic desensitization is due to a defective "grouping" of the anxiety-making situations. Such difficulty could come from the fact that the history of the illness, the metamorphosis of the symptoms, their successive masks, are unknown. In such a case psychoanalytical techniques could be helpful.

With the previous patient, the grouping of the anxiety-making situations was facilitated, simplified, clarified and certainly the desensitization was made easier by the psychoanalytical insight, the improved consciousness of neurotic automatisms, of their deep significance, of their origin, of the history of their fixation and transformations, of their repetitions, yet only analogical repetitions, which are inherent to them.

On this basis, other combinations can be suggested, for instance the help of psychoanalytical techniques during or after a particularly difficult desensitization. Here again, the synthetic use of the three methods could not only improve the results but also shorten the treatment, precisely because it would not be a simple addition but a synthesis. We can observe the same with systematic desensitization which is already synthetic to a certain degree. We must remember that, in true synthesis, certain properties of the isolated components are masked, while the combination sets off new qualities. Now, the question is: what qualities appear and what qualities disappear?

## RELAXATION, RELATIONSHIP, TRANSFERENCE, COMMUNICATION

Deep relaxation including eye and speech muscles excludes any emotion, any visual or verbal thought, a fortiori any transference and any communication from the subject. However he continues to feel, to perceive, to understand. The more he suppresses perturbing active operations, the more he opens his mind to the whole reality, to God as the mystics would say. Deep relaxation may be an indifference to small nothings, it is far from being sleep. What better "reinforcing of the ego" can we find?

To stick to the point, we must observe that systematic desensitization not only uses a lighter relaxation but, as well as that, it uses imagination of anxiety-making situations, which requires an eyeball muscular activity, and communication of emotions, requiring a certain speech muscular activity. I usually also ask where the patient feels tense, so as to be able to improve the relaxation there. In other words, a total relaxation isn't required as deconditioning means.

I would add that, in simple progressive relaxation, before and after the deepest stages of relaxation and at best before and after the properly called relaxation session, transferred emotions can be felt and communicated. It is this important modification--a lapse of time between relaxation, emotion and its communication--that I allowed myself to introduce into my first "didactic relaxation", done with Doctor Bovier by the method which Professor Ajuriaguerra prefers to call "dialogue tonique". Thus, in a certain way, it is possible to cumulate the benefits of both methods, the strictly called relaxation and a psychoanalysis based on bodily relationships (a very approximate way of speaking).

Shortly, thereafter I had the privilege of being provided with a second didactic relaxation by Doctor Edmund Jacobson and it is with emotion and with the greatest interest that I remember our talks before and after deep relaxation.

In fact, with the patient I cited, the analysis of bodily tensions felt during the lightest stages of relaxation and communicated after the session permitted a considerable increase of the psychoanalytical insight. In the same way I myself felt my didactic relaxations were an important contribution to my didactic psychoanalysis, as well as directly useful.

## FIRST INDICATIONS FOR A SYNTHETIC APPROACH

The best way of treatment is that which is both the most economical (this notion includes the expense of therapist studies) and the most useful to the patient.

To my knowlege even for the most classical methods such as psychoanalysis, progressive relaxation and systematic desensitization, we don't have any precise statistics concerning their results. We have even fewer on more recent methods, such as the afore-mentioned. Even if we did have such statistics, we would still have to weigh up which method to use, and in what way, in each individual case. To this we would add the difficulty pointed out by Wolpe: simple human contact, regardless of the method used, has in a high percentage of cases a strong and beneficial psychotherapeutical effect.

Nevertheless on this uncertain background we can pick out some faint orientations. Here I shall note a few of them following what I said previously concerning the synthetic approach.

1. Progressive relaxation should be envisaged when the pathological neuro-muscular tensions predominate, without forgetting the high frequence of tetany and the fortunate effects of magnesium-therapy in these cases.

2. Systematic desensitization (which is already a synthetic method) could be tried when it is difficult to obtain relaxation in anxiety-making situations.

3. The introduction of psychoanalytical techniques could be favorable in the case of forseeble or verified failure of both the former methods, particularly in the case of massive pathological transference or when an adequate grouping of anxiety-making situations is too difficult or impossible.

Personally, as far as I know at the moment, in many cases I would tend to begin by a trial treatment of systematic desensitization based on a not too brief preliminary progressive relaxation. Depending on the results I would tend either to increase relaxation or to introduce a more or less deep psychoanalytical investigation, not excluding the possibility of later returning to desensitization.

Yet therapy and particularly psychotherapy remains to a large extent an ART, and in art (as in science) it is advisable to beware of over-simplified sketches.

# TENSION AND ANXIETY

# EXPLANATION OF ANXIETY TENSION STATES

Pat A. Tuckwiller, M.D.

Consultant, Charleston Area Medical Center
Charleston, West Virginia

The purpose of this informal talk, as the title implies, is to explain to patients, their spouses, relatives, or close friends in small group sessions, the nature of their anxiety tension state. A brief review of anatomy is presented to better understand the symptoms. The most common symptoms will be enumerated. Next, the normal function of the autonomic (or automatic) nervous system will be explained. This then is contrasted with the malfunction of this nervous system resulting in muscular tightness, which directly causes most of the symptoms of neuromuscular tension. Finally, relaxation lessons are described using the Jacobson techniques as modified by the late Dr. Henry Dixon, the former professor of psychiatry of the University of Oregon. This method of explanation was mostly learned and copied in large part by me from Dr. Dixon. These relaxation lessons are used as an adjunct for teaching patients to get the feel of tight muscles, in contrast with letting go and being at ease. Other suggestions for treatment and coping are then made. Between each of the four parts of the talk, we stop and allow questions and comments by the patients or their relatives so that the usual group session lasts approximately one hour. Complete understanding of an anxiety tension state is considered just as crucial as is a patient's knowledge for good control of other illnesses, such as diabetes mellitus.

An anxiety tension state may be defined as exaggerated, delayed normal reactions, which occur at inappropriate times and without a direct cause and effect relationship which is obvious to the patient. This illness occurs most often in people with more than average intelligence, in persons who are usually in a rush, in those who take everything too seriously, in people who worry about what happened yesterday and who fret about what may happen tomorrow.

A nerve may be likened to a telephone wire. The message is carried by a tiny electric current. From the standpoint of function, a person has three types of nerves: (1.) the motor nervous system, over which a message goes from the conscious mind to muscles, resulting in action such as walking, (2.) the sensory nervous system, over which a message goes for example from a pinched muscle to the conscious mind registering discomfort, and (3.) the autonomic nervous system, which works automatically without any conscious thought continuously controlling functions of the body, such as the beating of the heart, breathing, peristalsis of the bowel, secretions of body glands, or the blinking of an eye. This system is controlled by a telephone center in the hypothalmus toward the base of the brain at a completely subconscious level. It is this system which misfires and sends ill-timed signals in the illness we call an anxiety tension state.

Now for a brief review of anatomy. (Please imagine that now each one of you in the audience is a patient, relative, or interested friend and that you are a layman with very little knowledge of anatomy or physiology).

The heart is located in the middle of the chest with lungs on both sides. The reason many people think the heart is on the left side, is that the apex or lower part of the heart is nearest the chest wall where it is most easily felt in the left chest. The esophagus is the food tube which extends from the throat down the mid-chest, behind the heart, and goes through the left diaphragm into the top or fundus of the stomach located in the area beneath the left diaphragm, under the lower left ribs. The stomach swings across the mid-abdomen and empties into the small bowel, which has many loops in the mid-abdomen. The small bowel empties into the colon or large bowel in the right lower quadrant of the abdomen. The large bowel ascends along the right abdomen (the ascending colon). It makes a sharp bend in front of the liver under the right lower ribs, swings downward and across the mid-abdomen, and then upward to the left upper quadrant (the transverse colon). It then makes another sharp curve behind and lateral to the fundus of the stomach, then down the left side of the abdomen (descending colon) to an S-shaped segment of the bowel (sigmoid colon), and then the rectum and anus (or outlet).

Next, let us enumerate the most common symptoms. There may be blurring of vision, lightheadedness, uncertainty in balance, pain in the back of the neck which extends to the shoulders, down the spine, and to the back of the head and scalp muscles giving an occipital headache. There may be a sensation of weight on top of the head, a tight hand sensation around the head, or a generalized headache. There may be a choking sensation or a feeling of a lump in the throat.

There is often a tight feeling in the chest giving the sensation of shortness of breath or air hunger, resulting in frequent deep sighs or over-breathing (called hyperventilation syndrome). Often there is palpitation or consciousness of heartbeat which may be rapid and either regular or irregular with premature beats which give patients the sensation of "skipped beats, flip-flops, or heart coming up in the throat". As a result of the tightness in the throat and chest muscles, patients often develop the habit of swallowing in a subconscious effort to relieve the tightness and in so doing, swallow an excessive amount of air (called aerophagia). Then after a meal, the air is compressed in the fundus or top of the stomach under the left diaphragm and left lower ribs. Then they may have sharp pains and if they think the heart is located in the left chest, conclude that they are having pains in the heart. Belching may occur and, if forceful, gastric juice normally containing hydrochloric acid is regurgitated into the esophagus with a burning pain called "heart-burn". This has nothing to do with the heart, except that it is located in the esophagus in the mid chest just behind the heart. If the air is not belched, it passes on into the small bowel where a mixture of air and liquid is carried along by normal peristalsis (or movement in the bowel), causing gurgling and rumbling noises. You may know the old poem:

> "I went to the Duchess's for tea,
> It was just as I thought it would be,
> Her organs internal, made noises infernal
> And everyone thought it was me!"

Then there is increased gas by bowel or flatus, "gas pains", most commonly under the ribs on the left, just below the stomach, and under the ribs on the right or over the sigmoid colon in the left lower quadrant of the abdomen. Also, there is alternating constipation and diarrhea, bowel cramps, and abdominal aching. This is often diagnosed as irritable bowel, spastic colitis, or mucous colitis.

There may be numbness and tingling or pulling sensations with aching in the arms and legs, cold sweaty hands and feet, or excessive sweating of the armpits. There are often burning, itching, or crawling sensations of the skin or numb spots over various spots of the body. Weak spells are common and generalized weakness or a sensation of weakness in the knees. Fatigue is common especially in the morning, even though one has apparently slept well. This is called chronic nervous fatigue or neurasthenia.

There are many more symptoms. I have merely reviewed the more common ones. Now, will everyone here who has had most of these symptoms at one time or another, please raise your hand?

How does the autonomic nervous system function normally? The central message control center in the hypothalmus at the base of the brain sends messages to the adrenal glands located just above each kidney, which responds with appropriate amounts of adrenalin secreted into the blood stream according to the need at any moment. Now, suppose that you go to see a circus parade and a lion gets out of his cage and heads directly towards you. That moment, the telephone message goes to the adrenal glands. A large amount of epinephrine is secreted into the blood stream. Then what happens? Your heart beats fast, you get a full feeling in the "pit of your stomach" and your muscles tighten up, but you can fight harder or run faster because of this extra adrenalin. But let us say they get the lion back in the cage and you need not fight or run. Nevertheless, after this severe scare you feel "all in". We call this "acute nervous shock" or "nervous exhaustion". But in a normal person, as soon as he is safe, the adrenalin flow which was too low after the scare adjusts back to normal average level and everything is all right. The same reaction may be normally evoked by anger, embarrassment, news of tragedy especially in ones' family, or even by elation. In all these instances, one doesn't worry about the symptoms because the cause is understood.

An anxiety tension state is usually the result of a gradual build-up over a period of many weeks, months, or years. This is so insidious and has developed so gradually that patients are not aware of their muscle tightness, which is translated into physiological somatic discomforts. The great Scotch poet, Robert Burns, in his poem, "Ode to a Louse", wrote these famous lines:

"Would the gift the Giver give us,
To see ourselves as others see us,
It would from many a foolish air and blunder free us."

Thus the need for relaxation exercises, so patients learn to feel the difference between tight muscles and complete muscle relaxation. An explanation will help you see the difference, but in order for you to learn control, you must be taught to feel the difference by repeated sessions thirty minutes each of tightening and letting go. You are requested to take leisurely strolls daily for at least an hour.

Now, let us return to the physiology of the illness. After this insidious onset of neuromuscular tightness, inappropriately-timed telephone messages go from the subconscious control center to muscles here and there, off and on, without any apparent cause. Now you don't understand the cause and naturally you are concerned. As a result, the tension mounts higher and higher and then you may have various reactions.

The four most common are: (1.) the development of fears or phobias, (2.) onset of chronic exhaustion or fatigue (usually worse in the morning), (3.) depression with crying spells, frustration, and even ideas of suicide, and (4.) shaking spells, tantrums, throwing things, or pulling your hair (called hysteria).

What are the causes of this build-up of nervous tension? Many! First, heredity plays a part. Many of us are born with the tendency. Next, childhood experiences are important. Trials, tribulations, illnesses, injuries, operations, trouble at home or work, financial worries all take their toll. A poorly-balanced program of living very often leads to this illness.

Finally, here are suggestions for what you must do to recover completely. It will take time, patience, desire, and determination. Medication--sedatives, tranquilizers, and antidepressants give only partial and temporary relief. These are helpful until you learn self-control. Then these should be gradually reduced and eliminated.

After you fully recognize muscle tightness and learn to release it, you must get the habit of practicing the art of relaxation. Then follows the most important prescription: A well-balanced program of living. This includes proper proportions of:

1. Work
2. Rest
3. Play
4. Religion

Overdo one or two of these and neglect the others, and you will again become tense and anxious. Remember you can overdo any good thing. Keep busy with a well balanced program of living and your life will gradually become more happy and meaningful. While it is all right to hurry occasionally, get out of the habit of being forever in a rush. Live your life one day at a time. Quit worrying about what happened yesterday or what might happen tomorrow. Quit crossing your bridges before you come to them.

Adopt the philosophy of Alcoholics Anonymous: "God grant us the serenity to accept those things we cannot change, the courage to change those things we can change, and the wisdom to know the difference."

Sir William Osler, often called "Father of American Medicine", in one of his many talks said something about as follows:

> "Heed the salutation of the dawn.
> Live your life in air-tight compartments, one day at a time."

He likened life to a great battleship, in the hull of which vessel are built many air-tight chambers. If a torpedo strikes the ship and water rushes in one compartment, there are enough air chambers left that the ship will stay afloat and on a fairly even keel. If you so live your life, you will keep it on a reasonably even keel.

My dear patient, while we counselors and physicians can do much to help you, the ultimate responsibility for your recovery is entirely up to you. Remember also, help is available from a Higher Power. May He help you to steer your course well on the tumultuous Sea of Life!

# EFFECTS OF PROGRESSIVE RELAXATION AND AUTOGENIC TRAINING ON ANXIETY AND PHYSIOLOGICAL MEASURES, WITH SOME DATA ON HYPNOTIZABILITY

Paul M. Lehrer, Ph.D., John M. Atthowe, Ph.D.

College of Medicine and Dentistry of New Jersey
Rutgers Medical School
Piscataway, New Jersey

B. S. Paul Weber, M.D.
The Carrier Foundation
Belle Mead, New Jersey

Autogenic training (Schultz and Luthe, 1969) and progressive relaxation (Jacobson, 1938) are two of the most widely used relaxation techniques. The two techniques have very different rationales.

Autogenic training was derived from observations on individuals who were undergoing hypnosis, and its rationale is to allow the body to reestablish a state of homeostasis. Although autogenic training usually involves attaining deeper states of relaxation, it also has been used to induce abreactive emotional discharges. Its focus is primarily on sensations of diminished sympathetic and increased parasympathetic nervous system activity. For example, autogenic training requires the subject to concentrate on such formula as "My arms are warm and heavy;" "My heartbeat is calm and regular;" "It breathes me" ("My breathing is automatic"); My solar plexus is warm;" etc.

Progressive relaxation, on the other hand, involves learning to recognize very faint sensations of tension in the skeletal muscles and learning to control muscle tension until the tension completely disappears. As described by Jacobson (1938, 1964), the technique uses very little suggestion. It is taught as a muscular skill, and is oriented to achieving very deep levels of muscular relaxation. Gellhorn (1958) has suggested a mechanism whereby very deep muscular relaxation may produce lower physiological activation in general, and Jacobson (1938) presents numerous case examples illustrating the effectiveness of progressive relaxation in treating a wide variety of psychosomatic disorders.

Davidson and Schwartz (1976) have suggested that different relaxation training techniques may have different effects on people, depending on the specific skills that are taught, the organ systems at which they are directed, and the parts of the brain that are most directly involved in the learning. This contrasts with the theory proposed by Benson (1975) that all relaxation techniques produce a single "relaxation response". Since the focus of autogenic training is more directly on the autonomic nervous system and on the smooth muscles than is that of progressive relaxation, Davidson and Schwart's theory would predict that autogenic training produces greater autonomic and smooth muscle changes.

Few comparative studies if autogenic training and progressive relaxation have been done. Shapiro and Lehrer (1979) found no heart rate or skin conductance differences between autogenic training and progressive relaxation, but did find that subjects given autogenic training reported more sensations of warmth and heaviness in the limbs than subjects in the relaxation group. Neither group differed physiologically from a waiting list control group, but both treatment groups reported a decrease in anxiety symptoms. A possible reason for the lack of physiological differences between groups was that the subjects were not screened for anxiety. Other research in our laboratory (Lehrer, 1978) had indicated that physiological changes produced by progressive relaxation can be measured among anxiety neurotics, but not among normal subjects. Similarly, Borkovec and Sides (1979) conclude from their literature review that more dramatic physiological findings in relaxation studies occur when highly anxious subjects are studied.

Another dimension along which progressive relaxation and autogenic training should differ is in the relationship of hypnotizability to treatment response. Because of the similarity of autogenic training to self hypnosis, we expected that response to autogenic training would correlate well with measures of hypnotizability. Progressive relaxation, on the other hand, appears to be much more analogous to direct muscle training or biofeedback than to hypnosis, since the procedure focuses on learning to discriminate and to coordinate subtle physiological processes, rather than learning to maintain a particular focus of attention. There is evidence that the ability of individuals to control their finger temperature by biofeedback is not related to hypnotizability (Roberts et al., 1965). Thus we did not expect measures of hypnotizability to be highly correlated with learning progressive relaxation.

## METHOD

### Subjects

Fifty-five male subjects were recruited from newspaper articles and advertisements inviting participation from anxious men interested in being taught to relax as part of an experiment. Potential subjects were sent the IPAT Inventory (Krug, et al., 1976), and only those who scored greater than 1 standard deviation beyond the mean of the normative group mean were accepted. This was the criterion used by Edelman (1970), in a study that did reveal physiological effects of progressive relaxation. We excluded all men who had previous experience with any form of relaxation training, men who were taking medication that could not be discontinued, and men who were suffering from hypertension, heart disease or epilepsy. Subjects stopped taking all medication long enough for it to clear their systems prior to both testing sessions. Based on their levels of hypnotizability, subjects were assigned to one of four experimental groups: Progressive relaxation, autogenic training, a false feedback control condition, and a waiting list control. Each condition had an equal number of subjects at each hypnotizability level.

## Testing Hearing and Hypnotic Susceptibility

The subject's first session at the laboratory included receiving a brief audiometer test and a test for hypnotic susceptibility. For safety reasons, subjects with measurable hearing loss were excluded from the study. Hypnotic susceptibility was tested via a modified version of the Stanford Hypnotic Susceptibility Scale Form C (Weizenhoffer and Hilgard, 1962). Three items of Form C of a dissociative nature (age regression, amnesia, and negative visual hallucation, were excluded, because they appeared to measure a kind of hypnotic experience of relaxation. Table 1 shows the scale that we used, including Hilgard's (1965) norms for the per cent of subjects passing each item. Unlike in Form C, the items were not presented in order of difficulty. We classified subjects as "high hypnotizable" if they passed 8 or more items which, according to Hilgard's norms, should include approximately all subjects scoring above one standard deviation from the mean of the population. For purposes of assigning subjects to groups based on hypnotizability, we classified subjects as "low hypnotizable" if they passed no more than 3 items, and thus included approximately all subjects scoring below one standard deviation from the mean of the population. All other subjects were classified as "moderately hypnotizable."

## Physiological Testing Sessions

All subjects received two physiological testing sessions, approximately five weeks apart. Subjects in the progressive relaxation, autogenic training, and false feedback conditions received their interventions between these two sessions. Each physiological testing session consisted of the following: First the subject was greeted and the measuring transducers were attached for heart rate, respiration,

Table 1. Items on the Hypnotic Susceptibility Scale

| Item | % Passing (Hilgard, 1965) | Order of Presentation | Order of Presentation in SHSS Form C |
|---|---|---|---|
| Hand lowering | 92 | 2 | 1 |
| Moving hands apart | 88 | 10 | 2 |
| Eye closure | 58 | 1 | * |
| Mosquito hallucination | 48 | 5 | 3 |
| Taste hallucination | 46 | 11 | 4 |
| Arm rigidity | 45 | 4 | 5 |
| Dream | 44 | 7 | 6 |
| Arm immobilization | 36 | 6 | 8 |
| Finger lock | 32 | 8 | ** |
| Eye catalepsy | 30 | 12 | ** |
| Anosmia to ammonia | 19 | 3 | 9 |
| Hallucinated voice | 9 | 9 | 10 |

*Included as induction only in Stanford Hypnotic Susceptibility Scale (SHSS) Form C.

**Additional items making up our scale.

and temperature from the surface of the dominant middle finger. Then the subject was asked to lie back in a comfortable reclining chair, and to relax as deeply as possible, with his eyes closed. He was told to expect five loud tones, but try to stay as relaxed as possible right through them. After five minutes of relaxation, subjects were exposed to 5 very loud (100 db) tones of 1000 hz and 1 sec duration. Thereafter subjects were asked to imagine a relaxing scene for 2 minutes and then an anxiety provoking scene for 2 minutes. The content of these scenes had previously been constructed in discussions with the polygrapher while the latter was attaching the electrodes to the subject. The content of the scenes was kept the same for both physiological testing sessions.

## Equipment

Physiological measures were recorded on a Beckman Type RM Dynograph. Heart rate was taken from standard EKG electrodes on the right arm and left leg, and was recorded through a cardiotachometer. Finger temperature was measured using a Yellow Springs thermister. Respiration was measured from the thoracic area via a graphite strain gauge transducer that was strapped around the body.

## Treatment Sessions

Subjects in the three groups other than the waiting list control group received four sessions of intervention. Training was given by medical students and graduate students in clinical psychology. Each subject in the three training groups was given four individual sessions. In addition, subjects were given written materials detailing their procedures for practicing. The progressive relaxation procedures were abstracted from Jacobson (1964), and the autogenic training procedures from Schultz and Luthe (1969). In the false feedback group subjects were instructed to relax quietly to try to clear their minds, and to try to recreate the feelings they had during the training sessions. All subjects were instructed to practice at home for two 20-minute sessions daily.

After each therapy session subjects were given a questionnaire to complete in which they indicated whether they had experienced any of a number of physiological sensations or thoughts that are indicative of anxiety, relaxation, or "autogenic discharges" (cf. Schultz and Luthe, 1969). In addition all subjects in the two "real treatment" groups and in the false feedback control group completed brief daily questionnaires in which they indicated the amount they practiced each day. They also rated their level of anxiety at their most anxious and most relaxed moments during the day and during their relaxation sessions on four 10-point scales.

## Psychometric Evaluation

Subjects were readministered the IPAT Anxiety Inventory approximately one month after their physiological post-test session. At this time, in order to assess expectancy effects, subjects were also administered a questionnaire about the extent to which they thought they had received "genuine" treatment.

# RESULTS

## Statistical Model

Analyses of covariance (ANCOVA's) were done on the Session 2 (post-test) minus Session 1 (pre-test) difference scores, with the Session 1 scores treated as the covariate, and treatment as a between-groups measure. For physiological measures, epoch or trial was included as a repeated measure. In all cases comparisons of progressive relaxation vs. autogenic training and treatment vs. control groups were also done.

## Physiological Measures

Heart rate. There were borderline significant differences between groups in maximum and minimum heart rate per epoch through most of the session (in the initial rest period, during the tones, and during the two imagined scenes). The comparisons between autogenic training and progressive relaxation (adjusted in the ANCOVA for first session heart rates) show that heart rates decreased significantly more in the autogenic training group than in the progressive relaxation group (Table 1). The discrepancy between the overall analysis and the autogenic training vs. progressive relaxation analysis may be explained by the somewhat higher within-group variance in the control groups. However, this heteroscedasticity was well within the limits suggested by McNemar (1962) for the valid use of the ANOVA, and may reflect less predictable emotional and physiological effects for the control conditions. Matched $t$-tests on change scores revealed significant heart rate decreases only in the autogenic training group. These differences are consistent with the hypothesis that various relaxation procedures have unique effect. One of the autogenic training formulas is, "My heart beat is calm and regular."

Finger temperature. No significant between-groups effects were found for this measure.

Respiration rate. No interpretable between-groups effects were found for this measure.

## Verbal Responses to the Treatment

Daily questionnaire measure. Figures 1 and 2 illustrate the marked differences between groups in the extent to which subjects practiced their techniques. The Treatment X Week interaction is significant for the number of days per week in which the subjects practiced, $F$ (6,88) = 2.20, $p < .05$; and for the number of minutes of practice time per week, $F$ (6,88) = 2.83, $p < .02$. Subjects in the progressive relaxation group increased in practice time during the weeks following each of the four therapy sessions, while subjects in the false feedback group decreased in practice time after the first two weeks. Subjects in the autogenic training group decreased in the regularity of their practice (days per week), and changed relatively little over weeks in total practice time. By the fourth week subjects in the relaxation group were averaging approximately one more practice session and an extra hour's practice time per week than subjects in the autogenic training and false feedback groups.

There were also differences between groups in the amount of anxiety experienced by subjects during their home practice sessions. The Treatment X Weeks interaction was significant, $F$ (6,88) = 3.24, $p = .007$, for subject's self rated anxiety at their most anxious point

Table 2. Covariance Adjusted Post-test, Pre-test and Heart Rate Change Scores

| Measure | Condition | | | | Overall Between Groups Effect | | Autogenic Training vs. Progressive Relaxation | |
|---|---|---|---|---|---|---|---|---|
| | Progressive Relaxation | Autogenic Training | False Feedback | Waiting List | $F(3,28)$ | $p$ | $F(1,27)$ | $p$ |
| Minimum HR/epoch | | | | | | | | |
| $\bar{x}$ rest period | .60 | -6.90** | -3.71 | -1.10 | 1.341 | <.28 | 5.659 | .025 |
| $\bar{x}$ before each of 5 tones | 2.88 | -5.76+ | -2.72 | -1.94 | 1.808 | <.16 | 8.424 | <.01 |
| $\bar{x}$ after each of 5 tones | 1.24 | -6.34+ | -4.00 | -3.05 | 1.396 | <.26 | 6.846 | .015 |
| $\bar{x}$ during relaxing scene | 2.48 | -5.72 | -2.51 | -2.26 | 2.296 | <.10 | 7.192 | <.015 |
| $\bar{x}$ during anxiety scene | 2.24 | -6.38** | -4.90 | -3.50 | 2.466 | <.08 | 13.144 | <.005 |
| Maximum HR/epoch | | | | | | | | |
| $\bar{x}$ rest period | -.13 | -6.68** | -5.38 | -2.64 | 1.293 | <.3 | 6.693 | <.02 |
| $\bar{x}$ before each of 5 tones | 2.58 | -5.84* | -3.94 | -3.46 | 2.199 | <.11 | 12.825 | <.005 |
| $\bar{x}$ after each of 5 tones | 1.90+ | -5.09*** | -3.26 | -3.76 | 1.445 | <.25 | 7.390 | <.02 |
| $\bar{x}$ during relaxing scene | 1.77 | -5.48+ | -3.47 | -2.99 | 1.498 | <.23 | 8.295 | <.01 |
| $\bar{x}$ during anxiety scene | .98 | -6.11** | -4.84 | -2.57 | 1.913 | <.15 | 10.669 | <.005 |

Significance of covariance - adjusted change scores (matched $t$-tests with $df = 14$):

+$p < .1$
*$p < .05$
**$p < .02$
***$p < .01$

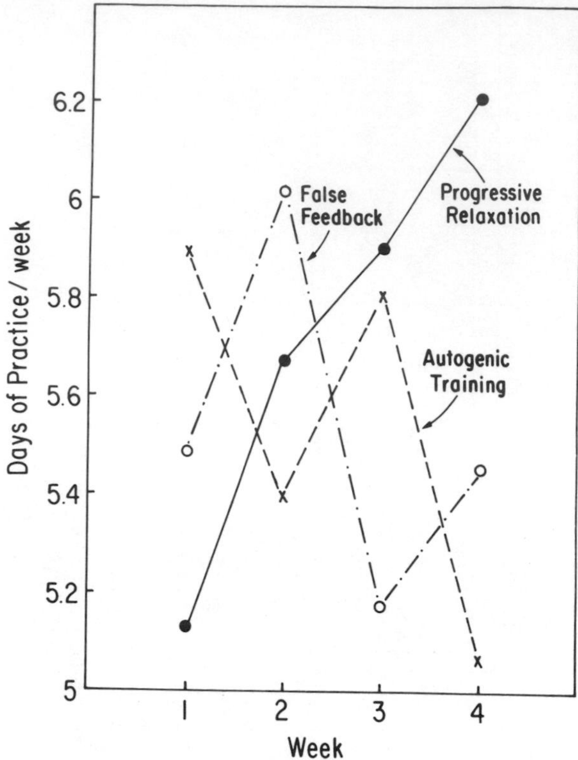


Fig. 1 Number of days per week of relaxation practice.

during their daily practice sessions. Figure 3 shows that subjects in the progressive relaxation group showed a steady decrease in anxiety over the weeks, and subjects in the autogenic training group showed a similar but smaller decrease in anxiety over the weeks; but subjects in the false feedback condition showed no change at all in this measure. There were no differences between groups in their ratings of average or peak anxiety during the day as a whole, or in their ratings of anxiety at their most relaxed moment in their daily relaxation session.

Questionnaire measures were given after each therapy session. Subjects were asked to rate a number of experiences they may or may not have had during each treatment session. The results for items that significantly discriminated between groups are summarized in Table 3. Subjects in the autogenic training group reported more sensations of heaviness and warmth in the arms (cf. the autogenic formula, "My arms are warm and heavy"), and more sensations of heart pounding than subjects in the other groups (cf. "My heartbeat is calm and regular"). The latter appears to be an "autogenic discharge" resulting from attention being focused on the heartbeat for the first time.

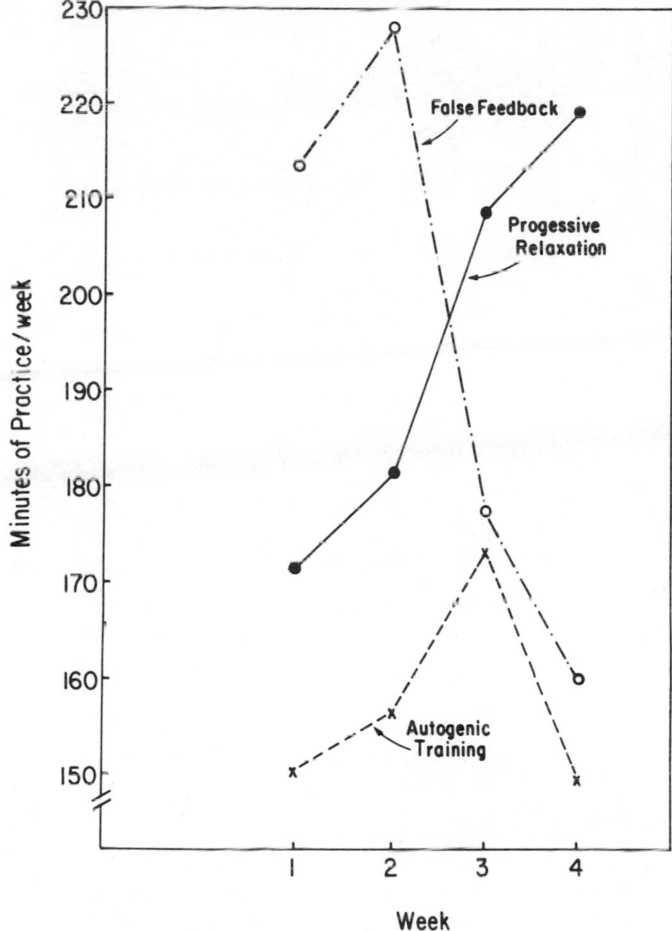


Fig 2. Minutes per week of relaxation practice.

That particular formula was given to subjects during the third training session, the only one in which there were significant differences between groups on this item. These findings are consistent with the theory that autogenic training has specific subjective effects. However, there were no differences between groups in subjects' perceptions of their breathing being calm and regular, or in subjects perceptions of their muscles being relaxed. Subjects in the treatment groups experienced more sensations of muscle twitching than subjects in the control groups, thus verifying the frequently made clinical observation that twitching often occurs during preliminary stages of relaxation in tense people. Increases in anxiety during training sessions was noted in the first session among the subjects in the false feedback condition significantly more frequently than among subjects in any of the other groups.

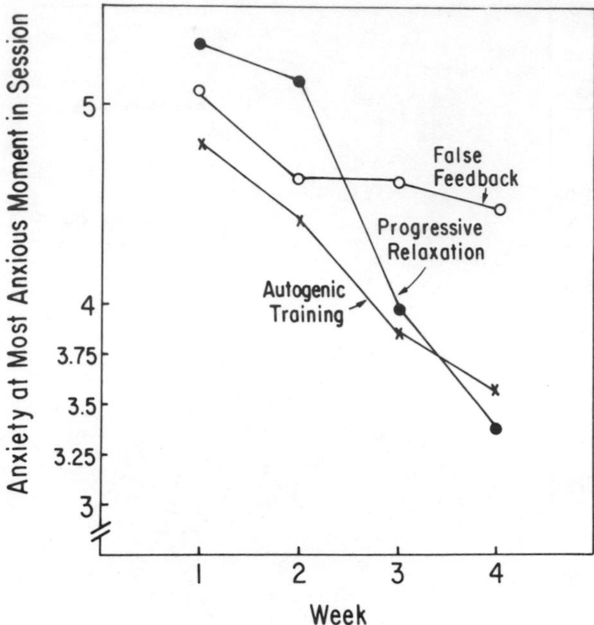


Fig 3. Self-rated anxiety.

FOLLOW-UP (ONE MONTH POST-TREATMENT)

IPAT Anxiety Inventory Scores

There was a significant covariance-adjusted main effect for treatment on the post-test-pre-test change scores of the full scale IPAT Anxiety Inventory scores. The treatment groups showed greater decreases than the control groups. The planned comparison ANCOVA showed that the treatment vs. control difference was significant at $F(1,43) = 9.126$, $p < .005$. There were no significant differences on the full scaled IPAT scores between the progressive relaxation and autogenic training groups. Matched *t*-tests on covariance-adjusted pre-test-post-test change scores revealed significant decreases for each of the treatment groups but not for the control groups. See Table 4.

Hypnotizability

Correlation coefficients were computed between hypnotizability scores and post-test-pre-test change scores on all physiological and paper-and-pencil measures, both within and across experimental groups. No consistent significant correlations were found. Also a median split was done on hypnotizability scores and, thus defined, a hypnoti-

Table 3. Per Cent of Subjects Reporting A Sensation During a Therapy Session

| Sensations Reported | Session | | | |
|---|---|---|---|---|
| | 1 | 2 | 3 | 4 |
| Warm hands | | | | |
| Progressive Relaxation | 37.5 | 37.5 | 56.2 | 56.2 |
| Autogenic Training | 43.8 | 93.8 | 100 | 100 |
| False Feedback | 33.3 | 33.3 | 46.7 | 60 |
| *P* | n.s. | <.001 | .003 | n.s. |
| Heaviness in arms | | | | |
| Progressive Relaxation | 62.5 | 75 | 75 | 62.5 |
| Autogenic Training | 93.8 | 93.8 | 100 | 100 |
| False Feedback | 46.7 | 46.7 | 40 | 60 |
| *P* | <.02 | <.02 | <.001 | <.02 |
| Pounding heart | | | | |
| Progressive Relaxation | 13.3 | 18.8 | 6.2 | 12.5 |
| Autogenic Training | 37.5 | 31.2 | 43.7 | 25 |
| False Feedback | 26.7 | 26.7 | 20 | 6.7 |
| *P* | n.s. | n.s. | <.05 | n.s. |
| Muscles twitched | | | | |
| Progressive Relaxation | 50 | 43.8 | 43.8 | 31.2 |
| Autogenic Training | 68.8 | 62.5 | 56.2 | 68.8 |
| False Feedback | 20 | 20 | 13.3 | 13.3 |
| *P* | .03 | .06 | <.05 | .006 |
| Anxiety increased | | | | |
| Progressive Relaxation | 6.2 | 6.2 | 6.2 | 6.2 |
| Autogenic Training | 18.8 | 12.5 | 6.2 | 6.2 |
| False Feedback | 43.8 | 20 | 20 | 13.3 |
| *P* | .03 | n.s. | n.s. | n.s. |

Note: *P* values are taken from $\chi^2$ tests.

zability factor was included in all ANCOVA's and ANOVA's. Again, no interpretable significant effects emerged.

## Belief in the Genuineness of the Instructions

At the time of the 1-month follow-up, subjects in the treatment and false feedback conditions had been asked whether they thought they had been given a "fake" relaxation procedure and whether this knowledge had affected their practice of or attitude toward the technique. (All subjects had been told prior to their giving consent to participate in the study that they might be assigned to a control group.) Chi square tests revealed no differences between groups on these questions.

Table 4. IPAT Anxiety Scale. Sten-Scores: Post-test, Pre-test Covariance-Adjusted Change Scores

| Group | Mean |
|---|---|
| Progressive Relaxation | -1.5* |
| Autogenic Training | -2.08* |
| False Feedback | -0.46 |
| Waiting List | -0.14 |

*Covariance-adjusted change score is significant at $p < .01$ using a matched $t$-test. The pretest score is the covariate.

## CONCLUSIONS

The autogenic training and progressive relaxation conditions both produced decreases in subjective ratings of anxiety with the progressive relaxation condition having a slightly greater effect. These decreases did not appear to have been produced by daily untrained relaxation (as in the false feedback condition) or by the belief in the "genuineness" of their techniques. Rather the effects appear to result from the specific training that had been given to subjects. In addition, as evidenced by frequency of reported practice, progressive relaxation appears to become more appealing to anxious people as they become more proficient in it, while autogenic training appears to sustain approximately the same level of interest from the beginning to the end of the first month of practice.

The physiological differences between groups were minimal. There was some evidence that autogenic training produced greater decreases in heart rate than did progressive relaxation. Since autogenic training specifically instructs people to slow their heart rates, these results lend some support to Davidson and Schwartz's hypothesis about the specific effects of various relaxation procedures. However, as in the study by Shapiro and Lehrer (1979), self report measures of anxiety were affected by both training techniques. Thus, although the physiological measures showed limited evidence of a general "relaxation response" produced equally by both techniques, the paper-and-pencil tests did produce such evidence. These results are consistent with Davidson's (1978) recent conclusion that specific effects of various relaxation techniques are superimposed on a generalized relaxation response. Perhaps more dramatic physiological effects would have been produced if we had used clinical diagnosis of anxiety as a screening criterion rather than response to the IPAT Anxiety Inventory. Research by Kelly (1976) strongly suggests that clinical diagnosis of anxiety is closely related to psychophysiological measure, while paper-and-pencil tests of anxiety are not and, similarly, Lehrer (1978) found decreases in autonomic reactivity produced by progressive relaxation training among clinically diagnosed anxiety neurotics, but not among nonpatients. Also it is possible that longer, more intensive training in relaxation may have produced greater physiological treatment effects. Borkovec and Sides (1978) conclude from their literature review that more lengthy treatment does produce more dramatic physiological effects.

The lack of relationship between hypnotic susceptibility and the various physiological and questionnaire measure of treatment-related change suggest that both autogenic training and progressive relaxation involve a form of skill acquisition that is not related to hypnotizability as measured by Stanford Hypnotic Susceptibility Scale items. It is possible that the Stanford Scale items were too difficult to adequately discriminate subjects who could learn to relax from subjects who could not do so as well. Indeed, the test begins with a relaxation induction, and it assumes that achieving relaxation is easier than achieving any of the other hypnotic effects measured in the test. Although the results of this study do suggest that the ability to learn to relax is unrelated to other hypnotic phenomena, it is possible that better prediction might be achieved by a test designed to measure lower levels of hypnotizability, or particularly to measure ability to do hypnotically induced relaxation. This is for future research to decide.

## REFERENCES


Barber, T. X., 1972, Suggested ("hypnotic") behavior: Trance paradigm versus an alternative paradigm, <u>in</u> "Hypnosis: Research Developments and Perspective," E. Fromm and R. E. Shor, eds., Aldine Atherton, Inc., Chicago.

Benson, H., 1975, "The Relaxation Response," Avon, New York.

Borkovec, T., and Sides, K., 1979, Critical procedural variables related to the physiological effects of progressive relaxation: a review, <u>Behav. Res. and Ther.,</u> 17:119.

Davidson, R. J., 1978, Specificity and patterning of biobehavioral systems: implications for behavior change, <u>Am. Psy.</u>, 33:430.

Davidson, R. J., and Schwartz, G. E., 1976, The psychobiology of relaxation and related states: a multiprocess theory, <u>in</u> "Behavior Control and Modification of Physiological Activity," E. Mostofsky, ed., Prentice-Hall, New York.

Edelman, R. I., 1970, Effects of progressive relaxation on autonomic processes, <u>Jnl. of Clin. Psy.</u>, 26:421.

Gellhorn, E. 1958, The physiological basis of neuromuscular relaxation, <u>Arch. of Int. Med.</u>, 102:393.

Hilgard, E. R., 1965, "Hypnotic Susceptibility," Harcourt Brace Jovanovich, New York.

Jacobson, E., 1938, "Progressive Relaxation," University of Chicago Press, Chicago.

Jacobson, E., 1964, "Anxiety and Tension Control," Lippincott, Philadelphia.

Johnson, R. F. Q., and Barber, T. X., 1976, Hypnotic suggestions for blister formation: Subjective and physiological effects, Am. Jnl. of Clin. Hyp., 18:172.

Kelly, D. H. W., 1966, Measurement of anxiety by forearm blood flow, Brit. Jnl. of Psychia., 112:789.

Krug, S. E., Scheier, I. H., and Cattell, R. B., 1976, "Handbook for the IPAT Anxiety Scale," Institute of Personality and Ability Testing, Champaign, Ill.

Lehrer, P. M., 1978, Psychophysiological effects of progressive relaxation in anxiety neurotic patients and of progressive relaxation and alpha feedback in nonpatients, Jnl. of Consult. and Clin. Psy., 46:389.

McNemar, Q., 1962, "Psychological Statistics," Wiley, New York.

Paul, G. H., 1968, Physiological effects of relaxation training and hypnotic suggestion, Jnl. of Abn. Psy., 74:425.

Roberts, A. H., Schuler, J., Bacon, J. R., Zimmerman, R. L., and Patterson, R., 1975, Individual differences and autonomic control: Absorption, hypnotic susceptibility, and the unilateral control of skin temperature, Jnl. of Abn. Psy., 84:272.

Schultz, J. H., and Luthe, W., 1969, "Autogenic Methods," Vol. 1 in, "Autogenic Therapy," W. Luthe, ed., Grune and Stratton, Inc., New York.

Shapiro, S., and Lehrer, P. M., 1979, Psychophysiological effects of autogenic training and progressive relaxation, Biof. and Self-Reg., in press.

Weizenhoffer, A. M., and Hilgard, E. R., "Stanford Hypnotic Susceptibility Scale," Consulting Psychologists Press, Palo Alto, Calif.

ACKNOWLEDGEMENTS

The authors are indebted to the following persons who served as relaxation trainers, polygraph operators, and data recorders: Richard Belser, David Lansky, Allan Shapiro, Gabrielle Sievering, Marilyn Bornstein, Stephen Josephson, and Roberta Itzkoff. The authors are also indebted to Alan Jusko for this technical advice and help.

This research was funded in part by General Research Grant #27-9817 from Rutgers Medical School. Computer time was made available by the College of Medicine and Dentistry of New Jersey.

# TENSION AND BIOFEEDBACK

# BIOFEEDBACK AND STRESS-RELATED DISORDERS: ENHANCING TRANSFER AND GAIN MAINTENANCE

Steven Jay Lynn, Ph.D., Judith Rhue, M.S. Candidate

Ohio University
Athens, Ohio

Robert Freedman, Ph.D.

Chief of Biofeedback Clinic
Lafayette Clinic
Detroit, Michigan

In 1973, it was proposed that..."a new behavioral medicine, biofeedback, may in fact respresent a major new developing frontier of medicine and psychiatry" (Birk, 1973). It is clear that if the promise of a behavioral medicine based upon biofeedback techniques is to be realized, effects generated in the laboratory or clinical setting must be shown to result in sustained modification or amelioration of various disorders. Thus, if a hypertensive individual has effectively learned blood pressure regulation in the laboratory or clinic, he should be able to maintain acceptably low levels at home, at work, in stressful situations, and in the presence of different individuals.

Indeed, it seems that a general assumption is that after sufficient biofeedback training, regulation of the target response will be as good without feedback as with feedback, and further, that treatment gains will be maintained across very different situations. Yet there are numerous reports that challenge these assumptions. That is, studies have shown that gains in the treatment of stress related disorders like hypertension, tension headache, and Raynaud's disease, may only be transitory (e.g. Lynn and Freedman, 1979). A number of studies also suggest that the regulation of the response learned in the training setting may be fragile, and easily disrupted by environmental events that generate the very responses the client is attempting to control (Holroyd, 1978).

The question which I will address in my talk is: How may we facilitate the long-term transfer of skills learned in the biofeedback training situation to situations outside the laboratory or clinic? Let us first examine the specificity and limitations of biofeedback treatment so that the rationale of the strategies and procedures that will be proposed will be brought into sharper focus.

While the traditional psychotherapeutic situation is far removed from the real world, the biofeedback environment is even more distant. That is, the biofeedback client is confronted with an impressive array of machinery in an atmosphere which encourages relaxation and turning out the "noise" of everyday life. This may reduce the likelihood of transfer outside the relatively constant, non-demanding, non-social biofeedback training situation.

Furthermore, the biofeedback paradigm typically ignores the specific physical, situational, and psychological antecedent stressors that may be essential to the production of a symptom (Mitchell and White, 1977). For example, a client with recurrent migraine headaches may be able to alter blood flow in the finger in the clinic, yet may not be able to exert self-regulation in a stressful job situation which is associated with the onset of headaches.

In a related vein, we may not observe treatment gains across various situations because symptoms may be reinforced by strong rewards or serve "secondary gains" associated with avoiding more aversive consequences than the symptom itself presents. In treating stress-related disorders like tension headaches with biofeedback alone, we ignore directly helping the client cope more effectively with aversive situations associated with the symptom.

One reason why gains may not be maintained over time is that non-specific factors or placebo effects associated with the impressiveness of the treatment and the enthusiasm of the therapist and client any result in only transitory symptom relief. If the treatment functions in part like other placebos, it is likely that treatment gains specific to such placebo effects will be short-lived.

The limitations I have cited suggest that it is essential for us to understand the causes and functions of a client's symptoms. A careful assessment may suggest the appropriativeness of specific interventions which might maximize treatment gains. After a thorough medical evaluation, further assessment is necessary. The etiologies of many stress-related disorders are often complex and multi-determined. Thus, an assessment of the client should include an evaluation of the cognitive, behavioral, and situational antecedents of the symptom, as well as the factors which tend to control, maintain, and possibly aggravate it. For example, if we find that a migraine headache is used by the client as a way of rationalizing an unsatisfactory social life, social skills training may be indicated.

Psychotherapy, relaxation approaches, and/or cognitive-behavioral approaches may assist the client in coping with identified problems, stressors, or situations which interfere with learning self-regulation or which may minimize such regulation across situations.

In weighing the potential rewards and costs of various treatment alternatives with the client, the clinician may opt to try relaxation or stress-management approach before embarking on a lengthy course of biofeedback training. For example, a variety of relaxation approaches have been used in the treatment of hypertension) including yoga relaxation exercises (Datey, Deshmukh, Dalvis and Venikor, 1969), autogenic training (Luthe, 1963), meditation (Benson, Beary and Carol, 1974), and combined relaxation and hypnosis (Deabler, Fidel and Dillenhoffer, 1973).

Various relaxation procedures have also been successfully used in the treatment of migraine and tension headaches, (Mitchell and White, 1977), Raynaud's disease (Jacobson, Hackett, Surnon, and Silverberg, 1973), and neuromuscular disorders. These approaches may be used where elevated levels of muscle tension or stress appear to mediate or exacerbate a particular problem. Clearly, if a client can learn to discriminate sensations linked with relaxation, such cues could be employed to help achieve control in a variety of situations (Budzynski, 1977). Such approaches may be particularly valuable for enhancing transfer of treatment effects with clients suffering from hypertension since elevated blood pressure is not so easy to discriminate as sensations associated with muscle tension.

Assuming that the client and therapist agree on a course of biofeedback sessions, what strategies and procedures may be used to maximize treatment gains?

In order to maximize the likelihood of transfer outside the training situation, it is important that a robust response first be obtained in the treatment context. If self-regulation is not demonstrated in the relaxed clinic or laboratory setting in the absence of feedback, it is unlikely that it will be evident in more demanding situations. If a response is not overlearned, it may be the case that it is easily disrupted by competing demands. In overlearning, learning is extended over more trials than are necessary to produce initial changes in the client's symptoms on the tartet response. Many sessions may be required before control is regular, consistent, and automatic both in the presence and in the absence of feedback. It is possible that some degree of symptom relief will be reported before the response is overlearned. Since clients with phasic disorders such as headaches and Raynaud's disease are more likely to terminate treatment when their condition improves, it is crucial that treatment extends beyond the point of initial symptom relief. Lengthy follow-ups are necessary in order to determine whether treatment effects persist and are not merely artifacts of placebo effects and/or the warning of symptoms associated with a phasic disorder. When treatment gains do not endure, evidence suggests that at least in some cases, additional "booster" sessions may reinstate physiological self-regulation (Budzynski, 1973).

Although I have emphasized the importance of overlearning, when a client rapidly develops a cognitive or physical strategy for control of a relevant response, additional training may not be necessary. The client should be encouraged to utilize whatever strategies are learned during training, in symptom-related situations. Meichenbaum (1976) suggests the use of films to show the client how other clients who have been successfully treated have learned to recognize the onset of symptoms and to use relaxation and coping strategies in key situations. Epstein and Blanchard (1978) have suggested using self-management strategies in which the client ultimately manipulates the events which influence behavior. The client is trained in self-monitoring the physiological response or symptom, is assisted in learning when to implement the self-control strategy learned during biofeedback, and instructed in self-reinforcement to maintain the practice of self-control.

Engel and Bleecker (1973) have suggested that "weaning the client from feedback" may enhance the perception of intrinsic cues and further the development of self-control. Such "weaning" may be accomplished by "fading the feedback." That is, first conditioning a robust response and subsequently gradually reducing or fading the feedback. Thus, after a response has been conditioned under continuous reinforcement, feedback may be gradually reduced to the point where the person is able to demonstrate adequate control both with and without the assistance of feedback.

Since the client must exercise self-control in everyday situations, introducing various stressors, distractors, and other real-life situations and stimuli in the treatment itself, may enhance transfer. Research in the area of neuromuscular disorders (Brudny et al., 1973), heart rate control in normals (Goldstein, Ross, and Brady, 1977; Shapiro, 1976), Raynaud's disease and EMG biofeedback assisted frontalis muscle control (Burish, 1978), shows that responses can be successfully established in stressful, atypical training situations. Another procedure which is as yet untested, is fading the feedback when the subject is exposed to stressful stimulation. If control begins to falter in the face of the stressor, feedback could be resumed on a continuous basis and again faded after an acceptable degree of self regulation is demonstrated.

This procedure could be continued until feedback can be completely withdrawn with no appreciable decrease in control of the response.

The use of multiple therapists may expand the range of stimuli in the training situation. Since the client must obviously maintain regulation in the presence of various individuals, this might enhance transfer. Varying the physical setting of the training may also facilitate transfer. With techniques of biotelemetry, it should be possible to monitor certain physiological responses in different settings and even provide feedback in such settings. An obvious extension of this approach would be to utilize inexpensive, portable feedback devices in the home and in the naturalistic environment. Relaxation procedures, autogenic training, meditation, and cognitive coping strategies are examples of some approaches that can also be "brought home" by the client and used as ancillary procedures where appropriate.

Certain factors inherent in the nature of various disorders may effect the likelihood of transfer of gains. Research thus far suggests that biofeedback is most effective in the treatment of disorders in which the response to be modified is easily observable, such as neuromuscular disorders, stuttering, or premature ventricular contractions. The neuromuscular disorder, for example, is generally present 24 hours a day, both inside and outside the laboratory. Its effects are usually readily observable without the use of external instrumentation. In contrast with tension headaches, which occur with varying frequency and very rarely in the laboratory, the neuromuscular problem is always available to be "worked on." The fact that neuromuscular disorders often have a clear physiological correlate (EMG activity) which is generally under voluntary control in normals, no doubt facilitates treatment with biofeedback. The tension headache, on the other hand, may not be consistently related to abnormal EMG or other physiological activity (Cox et al., 1975). Furthermore, regulation of muscle activity may simply be an easier task to learn than control of blood pressure, for example. Thus, certain conditioned EMG responses may be robust enough to be reproducible without the continued use of external monitors and in the face of the stresses and distractions of everyday life.

Up to this point, I have emphasized the need for careful assessment of the client and the inclusion of various procedures which may maximize gains. Clearly, biofeedback alone may not be a sufficient treatment for many of the complex disorders it is applied to. Yet it is not yet known when to employ the procedures I have mentioned, the sequence in which to use them, with whom and with which disorders they will work best, or the length of time necessary to teach them. Indeed, we do not yet know whether any of the suggested strategies alone or in combination will enhance treatment gains above and beyond biofeedback alone. And other approaches, like relaxation, may be equally effective and certainly less costly in the treatment of certain disorders such as hypertension. Clearly, a great deal of research is needed in which the use of transfer regimens is systematically manipulated with clients and normals and the outcomes carefully assessed over time. As in all other treatments, the efficacy of biofeedback and more costly transfer packages will be evaluated relative to available alternatives.

## REFERENCES


Benson, H., Beary, J. F., and Carol, M. P., 1974, The relaxation response, Psychiatry, 37:37.

Birk, L., 1973, Biofeedback: Furor therapeutics, Sem. in Psychia., 5:361.

Brudny, J. B. B., Korein, L., Grynbaum, L. W., Friedman, S., Weinstein, G., Sachs-Frankel, G., and Belandres, P. V., 1976, EMG biofeedback therapy: review of treatment of 114 patients, Arch. of Phys. and Med. Rehab., 57:55.

Budzynski, T. H., 1973, Biofeedback procedures in the clinic, Sem. in Psychia., 5:537.

Budzynski, T. H., 1977, Clinical implications of electromyographic training, in "Biofeedback Theory and Research," G. E. Schwartz & J. Beatty, eds., Academic Press, New York.

Burish, T., 1979, Generalization of EMG conditioned responses across different tasks and situations, Meeting of the American Psychological Association, New York.

Datey, K. K., Deshmukh, S. N., Dalvi, C. P., and Vinekar, S. L., 1969, "Shavasan": A yogic exercise in the management of hypertension, Angiology, 20:325.

Deabler, H. L., Fidel, E., and Dillenkoffer, R. L., 1973, The use of relaxation and hypnosis in lowering blood pressure, Am. Jnl. of Clin. Hyp., 16:75.

Engel, B. T., and Bleecker, E. R., 1974, Application of operant conditioning techniques to the control of cardiac arrhythmias, in "Cardiovascular Psychophysiology," P. Obrist, A. H. Black, and J. Brenner, eds., Aldine, Chicago.

Epstein, L. H., and Blanchard, E. B., 1977, Biofeedback, self-control, and self-management, Biof. and Self-Reg., 2:201.

Goldstein, D. S., Ross, R. S., and Brady, J. V., 1977, Biofeedback heart rate training during exercise, Biof. and Self-Reg., 2:107.

Holroyd, K., 1979, Stress, coping, and the treatment of stress-related illness, in "Behavioral Approaches to Medicine," J. R. McNamara, ed., Plenum Press, New York.

Jacobson, A. M., Hackett, T. P., Surman, O. S., and Silverberg, E. L., 1973, Raynaud's phenomenon: treatment with hypnotic and operant techniques, Jnl. of Am. Med. Assoc., 225:739.

Luthe, W., 1969, Autogenic training: Method, research and application in medicine, Am. Jnl. of Psychotherapy, 17:174.

Lynn, S. J. L., and Freedman, R., 1979, Transfer and evaluation of biofeedback treatment, in "Maximizing Treatment Gains: Transfer Enhancement in Psychotherapy," F. Kanfer and A. P. Goldstein, eds., Academic Press, New York.

Meichenbaum, D., 1976, Cognitive factors in biofeedback therapy, Biof. and Self-Reg., 1:201.

Mitchell, K. R., and White, R. G., 1977, Behavioral self-management: An application to the problem of migraine headaches, Behav. Ther., 8:213.

# TENSION AND STUTTERING

# ESTABLISHMENT OF FLUENT SPEECH IN STUTTERERS

Ronald L. Webster, Ph.D.

Director, Hollins Communications Research Institute
Hollins College
Roanoke, Virginia

Stuttering (or stammering, as it is sometimes known) is a distinctive form of behavior involving anomalous movements of laryngeal and vocal tract motor systems during attempts to produce speech. The repetition of sounds, syllables and words, the apparent "sticking" on a sound, and the blockage of voice during attempts to initiate speech are among the more discriminable physical features of stuttering.

Recent data support the concept that stuttering is essentially a motor control disorder typified by abnormally high tension levels in abductor-adductor speech muscles. Freeman and Ushijima (1975, 1978) conducted an electromyographic investigation using electrodes implanted in the intrinisic laryngeal muscles. During speech initiation, high levels of abnormal laryngeal muscle activity were found as well as clear disruptions in the normal relationships in abductor-adductor reciprocity. Freeman (1976) and her colleagues have also examined electromyographic data and simultaneous fiber optic films. Correlations were reported between the distorted activities of the vocal folds observed in the films and the disturbed electromyographic responses. In addition, Conture, et al. (1977) described vocal fold activity with fiber endoscope motion pictures of the larynx made during instances of stuttering. These investigators reported that sound-syllable repetitions were generally associated with the vocal folds being held in a somewhat abducted position. Folds were held tightly closed during instances of phonatory blockage. Abnormal abduction and adduction were observed during prolongation of sounds.

There is a developing body of evidence supporting the concept that stuttering is a physically based problem. The disorder has been found in all human language groups. Approximately one-half to one percent of any population of substantial numbers can be expected to demonstrate stuttering. Four times more males stutter than females. The time course in development is essentially the same from one group to another--approximately 95% of those who stutter do so by the age of seven. About one-half to two-thirds of the individuals who begin to stutter typically "outgrow" the problem by early adolescence. The disorder tends to run in families. Recent research on the familial patterns of stuttering suggest rather strongly that a set of factors transmitted from one generation to the other are responsible for the appearance of stuttering (Kidd, 1977).

In my laboratory, it has been observed that temporal patterns of phonatory activity are substantially different when stutterers are compared with fluent speakers (Bindewald, 1978). A computer system was used to measure each instance in which the voice was turned on while stutterers and fluent speakers read aloud a standard 500-word reading passage. Normally fluent speakers produced approximately one-half of their phonatory instances in the time window between 20 and 100 milliseconds. Stutterers, prior to their entry into our therapy program, showed approximately 25% of their phonatory durations within this same time window. At the end of the therapy program, the stutterers were similar to the normal speakers, showing approximately half of their phonatory instances within the 20-100 millisecond window.

Additional work conducted in my laboratory has shown that the voice onset characteristics of the stutterer are measureably different from those of the fluent speaker, even when the stutterer is producing fluent utterances of single-syllable words (Van Denburg, 1979). The initial pulses in the fundamental frequency of the stutterer's voice onsets were significantly larger in amplitude than those for fluent speakers, or for stutterers after they had completed therapy. This finding further supports the previous findings that the stutterer is abnormally tensioning the vocal folds during attempts to initiate phonation. Gable (1979) also found that voice onset times for stutterers during the production of unvoiced plosive consonants (p's and t's) were longer than those for fluent speakers. Once more, these data indicate that the temporal aspects of muscle contractions within the stutterer's speech apparatus are different from those of the fluent speaker.

Reaction time data also support the essential concept that stuttering has a physical basis. Adams and Hayden (1974) showed that voice onset and voice termination times were slower for stutterers than for nonstutterers. Speech reaction times slower than nonstutterers have been reported for stutterers by Starkweather, Hirschman and Tannenbaum (1976) and Cross and Luper (1979). McFarlane and Prins (1978) found that both speech and nonspeech reaction times were slower in stutterers than normals.

Factors that cause stuttering have not been reliably identified. The empirically oriented work cited previously in this chapter is all fairly recent in origin. The characteristic approach to stuttering during the course of the past 50 years has emphasized speculation, loose theorizing, and the reliance upon opinions of experts (Webster, 1977).

Travis (1931) attributed stuttering to defective hemispheric integration of information. Somewhat later, West (1936) advanced the concept of dysphemia. The central concept was that stutterers possessed an inherited predisposition for the breakdown of the central mechanism which controls speech functions. In some respects, stuttering was discussed as a variation on epilepsy.

Other investigators suggested that conditioned anxiety was the fundamental cause of stuttering. Johnson (1955) held that stutterers as young children were not clearly differentiable from nonstutterers. All children were thought to experience disfluencies in their speech as a natural corollary of language development. The response of adults to a child's stuttering was presumed to call attention to the child's speech and thus generate anxiety regarding speaking situations. Increases in anxiety were judged to be causal in the production of stuttering. Similar views were presented by Van Riper (1954) and Bloodstein (1958).

Numerous investigators have held psychoanalytically derived theories of stuttering (Webster, 1974). In general, this view held that the anomalous responses of stuttering were symptoms of an internalized emotional conflict. The stuttering behavior, per se, served to reduce the neurotic needs of those afflicted. The elaborate concepts in psychoanalytic thinking have had little real impact in facilitating developments in either therapy or research.

Learning theorists have also speculated about the possible origins of stuttering. Wischner (1950) suggested that reinforcement for stuttering could possibly be derived from reductions in anxiety occurring with the termination of the speech block. Sheehan (1958) presented a learning theory approach based on a double-approach avoidance conflict model similar to that previously described by Miller. Sheehan held that stuttering represented an oscillatory approach to speaking and nonspeaking based on the relative strength of the desire to speak versus the relative strength of the motivation to avoid speaking. Shames and Sherrick (1963) also presented a fairly straightforward learning based suggestion regarding the development of stuttering. These investigators considered the possible roles of positive reinforcement, negative reinforcement, and schedules of reinforcement in the development of stuttering, and indicated that these conditioning principles could support stuttering in children who occasionally showed disfluencies.

Unfortunately, theories of stuttering have suffered badly from the poor definition of concepts, the lack of parsimony in structure, and highly selective inclusion of empirical data. Recent advances in our knowledge of lawfulness in the observable behavior of stuttering once more emphasizes the merit of a strong empirical orientation in the development of scientific knowledge.

There is an emerging organization of empirical data that implicates the role of disturbed auditory feedback in the production of stuttered speech (Webster, 1974). The basic data involved in this view of stuttering all focus on specific empirical conditions that influence the speech characteristics of stutterers and/or normal speakers.

The delay of auditory feedback via special tape recorders reduces the fluency of nonstutterers and, surprisingly, enhances the fluency of the stutterer. Under conditions in which white noise masking is varied in intensity, the loudness of a normal speaker's voice can be driven up and down by manipulating the intensity of the noise presented to the ear. The stutterer shows somewhat the same effect, but when the white noise reached a sound pressure level of approximately 85 Db, fluent speech is generated. Other conditions that enhance the fluency of stutterers include whispering, rhythmic stimulation, singing, choral reading, and the adaptation phenomenon (Webster, 1974). The fact that these conditions have loci of effects at either the larynx or the ear suggests that there may be a working relationship between those mechanisms that process auditory feedback and those mechanisms involving the control of speech.

The concept of the servo mechanism has been applied to speech (Fairbanks, 1954; Webster and Lubker, 1964; Mysak, 1966). The basic idea is that the output of the servo mechanism (speech) is continuously monitored by a system that has stored within it a plan of the activities that are to be taking place on the output side of the system. Feedback of information about the output is compared with the plan and then rapid adjustments are made in the channels to control output and sustain it within predetermined levels. It is recognized that when the feedback signal is momentarily interfered with in servo mechanism, there is an abrupt increase in the level of output of the system. In effect, the system becomes momentarily underdamped and output characteristics are instantaneously distorted via overshooting.

It does appear as if there are mechanisms within the auditory system of the stutterer that may be responsible for disruptions in the transmission of a clear signal from the speech mechanism to the auditory mechanism. Specifically, it appears as if middle ear muscle contractions that occur in stutterers are somewhat different in intensity and timing relative to speech onset than they are in normally fluent speakers. In normals, middle ear muscle contractions occur approximately 60 to 100 milliseconds prior to the initiation of speech. In stutterers, during instances of stuttering, the middle ear muscles contract at the same time or slightly after speech is initiated. It appears as if the mistimed responses of the middle ear muscles interfere with the passage of auditory feedback into the auditory system. Interference in feedback in turn leads to momentary overshootings of the output producing the characteristic movements of the repetitions, prolongations and voice blockages characteristic of stuttering. This abbreviated version of the mechanism that may underly stuttering is described more fully elsewhere (Webster, 1974).

The essential point of all the information reviewed to date is that stuttering may be most parsimoniously considered as a muscle tension disorder that occurs intermittently during attempts to produce speech. The physical features of stuttering, the physical stimulus conditions that influence stutterers and fluent speakers, and the possible underlying physical mechanisms, all support the idea that therapeutic methods should focus tightly and carefully on empirical aspects of stuttering. The traditional emphasis on theory, the loosely defined therapeutic procedures, and the folklore of stuttering can progressively be replaced by scientifically derived approaches to the problem. In particular, a point to be emphasized here is that successful stuttering therapies might very well be expected to be derived from the careful, empirical analysis of the physical features of stuttering. The therapy program to be described below supports this point of view.

During the past 12 years my colleagues and I at Hollins College have developed the Precision Fluency Shaping Program, a stuttering therapy based on the systematic reconstruction of respiratory, phonatory and articulatory responses. Work on the Precision Fluency Shaping Program originated in response to the observation that traditional stuttering therapies were relatively ineffective in promoting fluent speech. The best inference that could be drawn from the literature indicated that about 25% of those cases staying in therapy for periods of from one to three years showed noticeable improvements in speech fluency. Data reported were often subjectively based and little quantification of stuttering was attempted. Consequently, it was difficult to assess the true levels of effectiveness in these therapies. The emphasis in the traditional approaches on attitudes, feelings and self-perceptions seemed to have little to do with the essential physical features of stuttering. We felt that it might be particularly useful to work on the development of a physically based, empirically oriented stuttering therapy.

The evolution of the Precision Fluency Shaping Program has been described elsewhere (Webster, 1980). In addition, the detailed structure of the program has also been previously reported (Webster, 1977). Over 1200 stutterers have now been treated in the three-week therapy program conducted at Hollins College. There are three segments to the therapy. Each of the segments ia approximately one week in duration.

Briefly, the first segment of therapy involves slowing speech down until it appears to be moving in slow motion. In order to accomplish this goal, syllable durations are increased markedly to specific temporal values. The purpose of the prolonged speech pattern is to permit the individual to observe details of speech movements while they are occurring. The establishment of the slowed speech pattern is followed by the careful reconstruction of respiratory responses. We have observed that roughly two-thirds of the stutterers we have seen demonstrate perturbed respiratory patterns. Given the fact that effective control of voicing (taught later in therapy) depends upon effective control of respiration, diaphragmatic breathing is established in therapy. Respiratory control is taught using a small biofeedback trainer that measures chest wall circumference changes. With the respiration trainer, it is possible to establish diaphragmatic control of breathing in a relatively short period of time. The new respiratory pattern is then generalized to settings outside the clinic.

The next step in the therapy involves the isolation of phonatory behavior. In particular, the client is taught how to initiate voicing with gentle onsets. This means that the client learns to produce a "functionally relaxed" voice onset characterized by initial low amplitude voice pulses that gradually grow to normal amplitude levels. The gentle onset target behavior is taught using a small computer device that measures physical properties of the acoustic signal during voice onset attempts, evaluates them, and then signals the results of the evaluation to the user. This device, the Voice Monitor, establishes precision control of the gentle voice onset target and facilitates the client's overlearning of the appropriate behaviors. The gentle onset target is practiced diligently with: (1.) vowel sounds; (2.) syllables beginning with voiced continuant consonants; (3.) syllables beginning with voiceless fricatives; and (4.) syllables beginning with plosive consonants. Basic tasks involved at this stage of therapy involve the coordination of the Gentle Voice Onset with the articulatory gestures that are typical of various phoneme classes in the language.

It is particularly important to note that all respiratory, articulatory activities have been defined empirically. Central values for all specific fluency skills and permissible variations have been established. It is important to emphasize the fact that the power of the therapeutic process for the stutterer seems to be linked directly to the precision and objectivity with which the critical response elements in therapy are defined. The physical definition of the behaviors at focus in therapy promotes client self-awareness of the responses that are basic to the generation of fluent speech.

During the second segment of therapy, the durations of syllables are reduced to near normal values, voice onsets are reduced somewhat in exaggeration, and respiratory patterns are further integrated with speech. Practice exercises involve using the fluency generating skills with short words, longer words, and then short self-generated sentences. Parallel transfer activities are included in all segments of the program that involve the use of fluency generating skills in situations outside the clinic workroom. These transfer exercises have been empirically identified and the inclusion on a parallel basis appears to be essential for the later effective transfer of fluency and its subsequent retention outside the clinic.

The last segment of the program involves the intensive transfer of fluency generating skills to settings outside the clinic. Clients begin this work by making short telephone calls and gradually extend their activities to complex conversations outside the clinic. By the time the client has reached the end of the 19-day therapy program, fluent speech has been transferred into a wide range of difficult speaking situations. Transfer of fluent speech into the client's home environment is normally a routine matter that is accomplished with relatively little difficulty.

The results obtained with the Precision Fluency Shaping Program are particularly encouraging (Webster, 1977). In one study conducted on a random sample of 200 treated cases, it was found that at the end of therapy 90% of the cases obtained disfluency scores in the range of the normally fluent speaker. In addition, self-report data derived from the Perceptions of Stuttering Inventory showed that 89% of the cases obtained scores similar to those of fluent speakers. The PSI score indicates the extent to which the individual will participate in or avoid various types of speaking situations.

A follow-up study one year after treatment showed that 70% of the cases sustained normal levels of fluency and normal scores on the Perceptions of Stuttering Inventory. Approximately 10% of the 200 cases had shown a slight regression toward pretherapy levels, approximately 10% showed a moderate regression to pretreatment levels, and approximately 10% were back at their pretreatment stuttering levels.

Table 1 presents a summary of data from several representative participants in the Precision Fluency Shaping Program. Speech samples were obtained from standard 500-word reading tasks and from conversations that were from 250 to 300 words in duration. The Perceptions of Stuttering Inventory total score (PSI) is judged to be in the normal range if the scores are 13 or below.

It seems clear that the development of a behavioral technology for the treatment of stuttering is attainable. As we have developed the program, we learned again and again that the precision with which response elements are defined and practiced by clients in therapy is

Table 1. Summary of Typical Stutterers' Speech Performance Data and Self-Report Scores Prior To and Following Participation in the Precision Fluency Shaping Program

| | | |
|---|---|---|
| Male, age 28<br>Pretreatment<br>Percent disfluent words<br>Reading = 42<br>Conversation = 36<br>PSI total score = 27 | After intensive three-week treatment program<br>Percent disfluent words<br>Reading = 0<br>Conversation = 0<br>PSI total score = 5 | Two years after the completion of therapy<br>Percent disfluent words<br>Reading = 0<br>Conversation = 0<br>PSI total score = 5 |
| Male, age 40<br>Pretreatment<br>Percent disfluent words<br>Reading = 45<br>Conversation = 80<br>PSI total score = 51 | After intensive three-week treatment program<br>Percent disfluent words<br>Reading = 0<br>Conversation = 2<br>PSI total score = 7 | Three and one-half years after completion of therapy<br>Percent disfluent words<br>Reading = 0<br>Conversation = 0<br>PSI total score = 5 |
| Male, age 9.5<br>Pretreatment<br>Percent disfluent words<br>Reading = 28<br>Conversation = 39<br>No PSI score | After intensive three-week treatment program<br>Percent disfluent words<br>Reading = 1<br>Conversation = 2<br>No PSI score | Three years and 10 months after completion of therapy<br>Percent disfluent words<br>Reading = 0<br>Conversation = 0<br>PSI total score = 1 |
| Female, age 6<br>Pretreatment<br>Percent disfluent words<br>Reading = no score<br>Conversation = 67 | Posttreatment<br>Percent disfluent words<br>Reading = no score<br>Conversation = 5 | No follow-up |
| Male, age 27<br>Pretreatment<br>Percent disfluent words<br>Reading = 18<br>Conversation = 23<br>PSI total score = 34 | After intensive three-week treatment program<br>Percent disfluent words<br>Reading = 0<br>Conversation = 2<br>PSI total score = 0 | No follow-up |

critical to the eventual outcome of the therapeutic process. The behavioral analysis required for the definition of the relevant fluency skills was a substantial undertaking and had to be completed prior to the codification of procedures for the therapy process. In addition, we are finding that whenever a training instrument can be introduced into therapy, the client has an easier task in therapy, the clinician becomes more efficient, and the overall level of learning attained by the client is more transferable into other environments than when noninstrument aided approaches are used. Finally, the intensivity of the therapeutic process seems to be of substantial importance in determining the quality of outcome. We have found that anytime the therapy program is used on a schedule which reduces client participation to below approximately 10 hours a week, progress in therapy is retarded and therapy dropout rates increase substantially. One implication is that many of the behavior reconstruction procedures that are used with speech problems (as well as other disorders) may suffer not so much from deficiencies in the basic technologies, but in deficiencies in their application.

## REFERENCES

Adams, M. R., and Hayden, P., 1976, The ability of stutterers and nonstutterers to initiate and terminate phonation during production of an isolated vowel, Jnl. of Speech and Hear. Res., 19:290.

Bindewald, R., 1978, "Phonation Times in Stuttered Speech: Before and After a Fluency Shaping Program," Masters thesis, Hollins College, Virginia.

Bloodstein, O., 1969, "A Handbook on Stuttering," Easter Seal Society, Chicago.

Conture, E., McCall, G., and Brewer, D., 1977, Laryngeal behavior during stuttering, Jnl. of Speech and Hear. Res., 20:661.

Cross, D. E., and Luper, H. L., 1979, Voice reaction time of stuttering and nonstuttering children and adults, Jnl. of Fluency Dis., 4:59.

Fairbanks, G., 1954, Systematic research in experimental phonetics. I. A theory of the speech mechanism as a servosystem, Jnl. of Speech and Hear. Dis., 19:133.

Freeman, F., and Ushijima, T., 1975, Laryngeal activity accompanying the moment of stuttering: a preliminary report of EMG investigations, Jnl. of Fluency Dis., 3:36.

Freeman, F., and Ushijima, T., 1978, Laryngeal muscle activity during stuttering, Jnl. of Speech and Hear. Res., 3:538.

Gabel, P., 1979, "Altered Durations of Stutterers' Initial /T/ After the Hollins Precision Fluency Shaping Program," Masters thesis, Hollins College, Virginia.

Johnson, W., 1955, "Stuttering in Children and Adults," University of Minnesota Press, Minneapolis.

Kidd, K., 1977, A genetic perspective on stuttering, Jnl. of Fluency Dis., 2:259.

McFarlane, S. C., and Prins, D., 1978, Neural response time of stutterers and nonstutterers in selected oral motor tasks, Jnl. of Speech and Hear. Res., 21:768.

Mysak, E. D., 1966, "Speech Pathology and Feedback Theory," Thomas, Springfield, Illinois.

Shames, G. H., and Sherrick, C. E., 1963, A discussion of nonfluency and stuttering as operant behavior, Jnl. of Speech and Hear. Dis., 28:3.

Sheehan, J., 1958, Conflict theory of stuttering, in "Stuttering: A Symposium," J. Eisenson, ed., Harper & Row, New York.

Starkweather, C., Hirschman, P., and Tannenbaum, R. S., 1976, Latency of vocalization onset: stutterers versus nonstutterers, Jnl. of Speech and Hear. Res., 19:481.

Travis, L. E., 1931, "Speech Pathology," Appleton, New York.

Van Denburg, E. J., 1979, "Wave Form Analysis of Stuttered Speech Before and After Completion of a Fluency Shaping Program," Masters thesis, Hollins College, Virginia.

Van Riper, C., 1954, "Speech Correction: Principles and Methods," Prentice-Hall, Englewood Cliffs, N.J.

Webster, R. L., 1974, A behavioral analysis of stuttering: treatment and theory, in "Innovative Treatment Methods in Psychopathology," Calhoun, K., Adams, H., and Mitchell, K., eds., John Wiley & Sons, New York.

Webster, R. L., 1980, Evolution of a target based behavioral therapy for stuttering, in "Proceedings of the First Annual Conference on Stuttering," D. Rosenfield, ed., Baylor College of Medicine, Houston, in press.

Webster, R. L., and Lubker, B. B. , 1968, Interrelationships among fluency producing variables in stuttered speech, Jnl. of Speech and Hear. Res., 11:754.

Webster, R. L., 1977, The establishment of fluent speech through the functional relaxation of vocal movements in stutterers, in "Tension Control: Proceedings of the Third Meeting of the American Association for the Advancement of Tension Control," F. J. McGuigan, ed., American Association for the Advancement of Tension Control, Louisville.

West, R., Is stuttering abnormal? 1936, Jnl. of Abn. Psych., 31:76.

Wischner, G. J., 1950, Stuttering behavior and learning: a preliminary theoretical formulation, Jnl. of Speech and Hear. Dis., 15:324.

# PRINCIPLES AND APPLICATIONS OF TENSION CONTROL

# PRINCIPLES OF SCIENTIFIC RELAXATION

F. J. McGuigan, Ph.D.

Executive Director, AAATC
Research Professor
Director, Performance Research Laboratory
University of Louisville
Louisville, Kentucky

The stresses of the modern world produce states of muscular overtension which in turn can wreak havoc on various systems of the body. The omnipresence of tension disorders in our society well attests to the fact that few people completely cope with tension problems of everyday living. Indeed, tension disorders are more common than the common cold, and they constitute unique problems for many professional fields. Consequences of a lifetime of excessive and unwise muscle tension are manifested in such pathological conditions as hypertension, coronary heart disease, colitis with attendant constipation and diarrhea, anxiety, excessive fatigue, bruxism, and headaches. The best answer to the question of how to wisely control the body and thus prevent or eliminate such tension conditions is in the effective application of progressive relaxation.

## SCIENTIFIC NATURE OF TENSION AND RELAXATION

An initial problem is the diversity of definitions for the terms "relaxation" and "tension". "Relaxation" can mean anything from a vacation to going on a picnic, while the meanings of "tension" vary widely from connotations of a hostile atmosphere to problems that are "solved" with alcohol. However, the classical, scientific definitions of these terms have to do with states of the skeletal musculature: <u>Tension is the contraction (shortening) of skeletal muscle fibers</u> and <u>relaxation is the lengthening of muscle fibers.</u> When we are tense, we contract our muscles and when we relax we "let our muscles go".

The consequences of these simple, straightforward, scientific definitions are enormous.

## PRINCIPLES OF PROGRESSIVE RELAXATION

An understanding of progressive relaxation properly begins with the everyday term "rest". Being from the vernacular, "rest" is not, of course, precisely defined, but it most assuredly has much value. The hard driving, high achieving scientist Ivan Pavlov found rest very valuable as a break from his daily routine. This fact may help to account for the longevity (86 years) of this vigorously active and productive man. His outstanding student, W. Horsley Gantt, has similarly practiced rest quite effectively, as perhaps is also attested to by his longevity, presently that of 87 years. Gantt continues to be among the most productive men I know, far more productive than the typical young scientist who has just left graduate school.

As valuable as rest is, it is still not maximally effective, nor is it always achieved. Progressive relaxation may be viewed as an improvement on this activity. The physician has long known the value of rest and has often prescribed it, frequently even "bedrest". As my medical school students have come to appreciate, however, mere prescription is not sufficient, for the patient still doesn't know _how_ to rest. At the conclusion of their progressive relaxation course when they state that they now know not only the value of rest for their patients (and for themselves), but _how_ to help them relax as well, by means of progressive relaxation. How much better, they have commented, is a prescription to relax than a prescription for Valium.

However, the task of learning to thoroughly relax one's muscles is not an easy one. There are some 1,030 separate striated muscles in the human body (which comprise almost half of our body weight). A lifetime of injudicious use of these muscles can lead to chronic malfunction of various bodily systems, for which there is no quick and easy cure. Just as we have spent our lives learning how to systematically misuse our muscles, it is reasonable to expect that many years are required to reeducate them. More is required than quick and easy cures offered by hypnotism, drugs, some popular "experts", or suggestive religions. It simply takes time and practice to patiently learn to reverse longstanding maladaptive muscular habits. Fortunately cultivation of a state of bodily rest can be achieved in much less time than it took to learn to misuse the muscles in the first place.

In learning progressive relaxation, one must cultivate sensitive observations of the internal sensory world equal to our natural ability to observe the external environment. In acquiring heightened internal sensory observation, one employs two simple, straightforward, physiological principles: (1.) Learn to recognize ("observe") a state of tension, and (2.) Contrast that tension sensation with the state of elimination of tension (relaxation). Each of the major muscle groups is then systematically tensed so that the learner can identify the unique tension sensation (control signal) for that muscle group.

And it is emphasized to the learner that he or she was the one who successfully eliminated the tension--not the instructor. Progressive relaxation puts the emphasis on the learner, not the teacher.

The tension sensation, incidentally, is called "the control signal" because it is literally a control for neuromuscular circuits, as diagrammed in Figure 1. Just as one learns to drive an automobile or a jet airplane by means of an accelerator, one can control the human body by means of the skeletal muscles. Let us see in greater detail just how this control of the human body is exercised.

When a muscle contracts (tenses), tiny receptors embedded in the muscle (called muscle spindle receptors) are activated. The activation of these receptors generates volleys of neural impulses that are carried to the brain along sensory control fibers. It is this muscle neural phenomenon--the generation and transmissions of neural impulses--that constitutes the control signal, the local sign of tension. This phenomenon was reported in 1842 by the emminent physiologist Sir Charles Bell, and has since been referred to as "the muscle sense of Bell".

By learning internal sensory observation one can become quite proficient in recognizing ("observing") these control signals wherever they may occur throughout the skeletal musculature. The long range goal of progressive relaxation is to achieve a state in which the body automatically monitors all of the control signals, instantaneously, and automatically relieves tensions that are not desired. Achievement of this state of habitual monitoring and automatic relaxing may take many years of sustained practice, though somewhat proficient stages of tension control might be acquired within weeks or months.

The complete process by which we can control our tensions is further illustrated by means of the closed loops at the bottom of Figure 1. Once muscles contract, generating volleys of neural impulses that are directed to the brain, there are complex central nervous system events; following this, neural impulses return by motor control fibers to the muscles. These complex circuits, involving muscles-small nerves-brain-small nerves muscles, are referred to as neuro-muscular circuits. By relaxing the skeletal muscles a state of tranquility is brought to all of the components of these neuromuscular circuits, including the brain inself.

To emphasize the importance of neuromuscular circuits, within which there are complex interactions between the brain and the muscles, that the concept of such circuits is not new--it is a venerable idea dating from the period of the early Greeks. Its evolution can be traced further through the writings of early philosophers, and then through the scientific renaissance in the research of physiologists and psychologists. Some of our most prominent thinkers in history have recognized that the human body functions in terms of

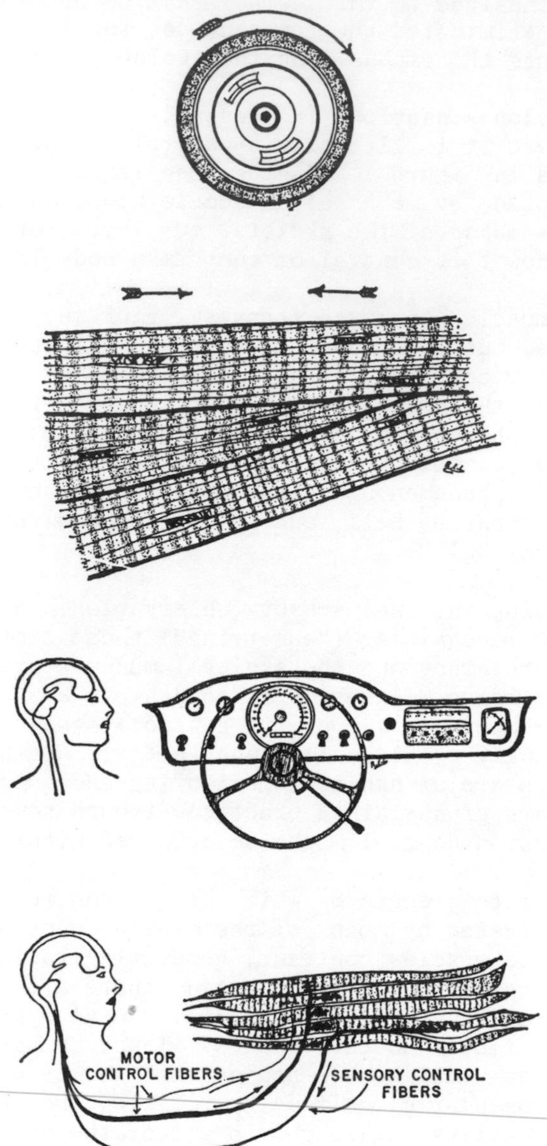


Fig. 1. Self-Operations Control. You run your car by manipulating the controls on and near the dashboard, whereby you make the wheels move at the rate and in the direction you desire. Likewise, you can run yourself by going on and off with the power in the controls which lie in your muscles, whereupon your muscles contract and relax in the patterns which suit your effort-purposes. Copyright by National Foundation for Progressive Relaxation, 1964, Jacobson, Edmund. "Self-Operations Control." 1964. Page 2. Reprinted by permission.

"messages" sent between the muscular systems and the brain. Perhaps the most popular presentation of this circuit concept was by Norbert Wiener in his well known book "Cybernetics." More than anyone before him, Wiener developed the notion that the body functions according to the engineering principles of feedback circuits in which information is conveyed from one region of the body to the other within loops.

Our question is: what is the controlling system within a neuromuscular loop? The answer was given quite clearly in the last century by the famous psychologist Alexander Bain--the only system over which a person has direct control is the skeletal muscular system. The "skeletal muscular system" has been synonomously referred to as the "voluntary muscles" precisely for this reason, i.e., when one wishes to perform an act, one moves the limbs or hands of the body by systematically contracting and relaxing the skeletal muscles. For instance, if I wish to go outdoors, I commence by putting one foot in front of the other. This point is so obvious that it does not need elaboration. What is not so obvious is that internal functions of the body are similarly controlled by means of the skeletal muscles. If you wish to increase your pulse rate you need merely tense the muscles of your body, as a simple demonstration during this reading will indicate. Conversely, once you have elevated your pulse rate, you can slow it again by decreasing the excessive tension you have caused by stiffening the limbs, the neck, etc. The essence of our message is to apply these principles to the more subtle functions of the body--to recognize that subtle, covert functions of the body can be controlled through slight muscle tensions.

But just how do you control bodily functions through systematic tensing and relaxing of the skeletal muscles? With even slight muscle contractions (tensions), the small muscle spindle receptors imbedded in the muscles are activated. Minimal volleys of sensory neural impulses directed to the brain can be detected as very subtle "tension" or "control" signals. It is with these extremely subtle signals that we can learn to control the activities of the body. More particularly, by learning tension control, we can control bodily functions in everyday life. The mechanism is through neuromuscular circuits that function as what engineers call feedback circuits or servo loops.

In considering just how you can use your controls, it may be of some value to recognize that there are different kinds of control systems in the world. For instance, consider the control switch for the power in the circuits that bring light into your room. When one works to throw a toggle switch up, power flows through the circuit and lights go on. Conversely, when one works to throw the toggle switch down, power ceases and the lights terminate. Are the controls in the muscles analogous to those of the toggle switch?

A little reflection answers the question in the negative. The point is an extremely important one for the learner of tension control: In activating the toggle switch, you must work to terminate power, to turn off the lights. Muscles, however, do not function in this way. To relax, you cannot work (force) the muscles to terminate power in the body. One cannot work (try, exert effort) in order to relax.

Now consider another kind of control--the accelerator on an automobile--a more appropriate analogy for muscle functioning. When you want the power on, you work. You expend effort to depress the accelerator, whereupon power flows. Conversely, when you wish to terminate power ("power off"), you ease up on the accelerator. You merely let go, and the automobile eventually comes to a halt. In short, when you want to perform an act, you must "press the accelerator" of the body (tense the muscles and let power "flow"), but when you want to establish a tranquil state of the body (relax), you merely let the power off--let go the muscles. In learning to relax you must learn how to properly use your muscular controls, the controlling elements in neuromuscular circuits.

In short, in each muscle sets of neurons (small nerves) conduct signals (messages) by means of sensory neural impulses to the brain for central processing, and there are also sets of neurons that carry motor messages from the brain to produce systematic contractions in the muscles. These neural and muscular events are quite well understood by physiologists. Science has accumulated knowledge of a sophisticated set of principles which explain how electrical, chemical, and mechanical events occur in muscles. For instance, we know that these circuits function very rapidly, neural impulses being conducted at a rate of some 40-100 yards per second in the human. An implication of this is that we can thereby exert very rapid control over the functions of our body, including the subtle covert functions that form major problems of individuals who seek to solve their tension maladies.

## GENERALIZED VS. LOCALIZED TENSION

In addition to localized tension (that confined to specific muscle groups) the body also generates a more generalized, widespread kind of tension which is carried chronically throughout the skeletal musculature. This general tension is a residual tension in which there is fine continuous contraction of the muscle fibers, along with a slight localized movements. Localized relaxation allows us to relax a particular, limited group of muscles, but a different technique is required for general tensions. Jacobson has also developed an effective procedure for controlling this widespread phenomenon. That technique is to very gradually and uniformly stiffen an entire limb and then gradually relax it over an extended period of time. This procedure, with sufficient practice, can allow an individual to relax the tension down to a zero level (which we can objectively measure through electromyography down to a tension level of zero microvolts). Needless to say, the untrained are not directly aware of either localized or generalized tension.

This reference to long term relaxation of generalized tension, incidentally, provides us with an opportunity to comment on several connotations of the term "progressive relaxation". First, an hour of continuous practice (performed daily) is necessary in order to progressively relax--or "get at"--the generalized tension in the major muscles of the body; this is continuous, progressive reduction of generalized, residual tension. Secondly, the term "progressive relaxation" indicates that during the practice period different muscle groups throughout the body are progressively relaxed--first one group, then another. And finally, one progressively tends toward a state in which you can automatically become tranquil throughout the entire body.

## TOTAL VS. DIFFERENTIAL RELAXATION

When we were first organizing the American Association for the Advancement of Tension Control, some delegates suggested the substitution of "reduction" for "control" in the title. This change would have been misleading because we do not advocate that the human race become vegetables. The term "tension control" is thus to be contrasted with "tension reduction." You simply could not function in life without tensions. The problem is not to eliminate tensions, but to control them so that they can be wisely used. In driving an automobile, you depress the accelerator and steer, but it is not necessary to excessively grip the wheel, to grit the teeth, to hunch forward, and to attempt to wear out the horn. Those who are untrained in relaxation continue to overtense in such ways until they complain of a stiff neck, a headache or being exhausted. These are unnecessary tensions. The primary purpose is to drive the automobile, and it does not help to simultaneously try to wear out the body. An efficiently-run (and thus well trained) person automatically relaxes all of the muscles which are not required for the act being performed, having learned to unconsciously recognize control signals for unnecessarily contracted muscles and to relax those tensions away.

In short, the wise have learned to selectively (differentially) relax those muscles not required for the act being performed. Consequently they do not become frustrated at the driver in front, honk, curse, or grit their teeth. You simply do not drive an automobile with your teeth. Rather, you differentially relax, which we define as the process of contracting only those muscles necessary for carrying out the purpose at hand, while relaxing all others in the body.

A dentist, for instance, spends many hours each day standing and bending over patients. Such an act requires considerable energy expenditure and one should learn to do it with minimum cost to the body. One can learn to stand and to bend in an efficient manner, using only those muscles required for treating the patient. Many people waste considerable energy by excessively tensing, even when they only stand or sit.

For the greatest benefit of society, Dr. Edmund Jacobson advocated the teaching of progressive relaxation to children, who, incidentally, acquire the skills more efficiently and more rapidly than do adults. If acquired early, children are then equipped to automatically and habitually employ the technique throughout their entire lives. Great advances in preventive medicine and clinical psychology could be achieved by so educating our young. Such progress comes slowly, but just as civilized society only recently learned to brush teeth and bathe regularly, perhaps we will eventually learn to differentially relax automatically, 24 hours a day.

In summary, tension is the contraction of skeletal muscle fibers, and relaxation is the elongation of skeletal muscle fibers. In order to acquire tension control, you need to first learn to recognize tension, and secondly, to let go the tension, relaxing it away. You then contrast that state of relaxation with the previous state of tension, recognizing that you thereby controlled tension on that specific region of the body. By exercising tension control you can orchestrate the skeletal muscle component of neuromuscular circuits in order to run your body for optimal benefit. The skeletal musculature can thereby be used to effectively control your obvious behavior, as well as more subtle functions of the body like the cardiovascular system and even mental processes. Efficient control comes from learning to differentially relax which is the process of contracting only those muscles necessary for carrying out your immediate purpose--all other skeletal muscles of the body should be relaxed. With sufficient practice you can achieve automaticity, a state in which the body automatically differentially relaxes, 24 hours a day.

With these understandings of the basic principles of scientific relaxation, let us apply them to our everyday living so that we can better learn how to spend the body's limited energy supply wisely.

REFERENCES

Jacobson, E., 1964, "Self-operations Control," Lippincott, Philadelphia.

McGuigan, F. J., 1978, "Cognitive Psychophysiology--Principles of Covert Behavior," Prentice-Hall, Englewood Cliffs, N.J.

# TENSION CONTROL METHODS IN PRIMARY HEALTH CARE

Galen Ives, B.Sc., M.Sc., M.B.Ps.S.

Department of Psychological Medicine
Barnsley District General Hospital
Barnsley, England

## ABSTRACT

Tension control methods would be expected to be especially appropriate in a primary health care setting. The paper reports the result of a pilot study in which a clinical psychologist visited two group practices in Sheffield for one session each per week over a two-year period. Patients were referred directly by the general practitioners and treated on the doctors' premises. Treatment methods included biofeedback, relaxation training and behavioral procedures.

Of those completing therapy 72 per cent made satisfactory progress. In the three months after termination of treatment patients made significantly less visits to the surgeries (36 per cent less) and received significantly fewer prescriptions for psychotropic drugs (50 per cent less) than in the three months prior to referral ($p<0.00001$ for both changes). These changes were maintained one year later in the three month period 12 to 15 months after discharge. Implications for future research are discussed and a brief description of a four-year project which is just beginning is given.

## INTRODUCTION

In recent years a number of surveys have attempted to estimate the prevalence of psychological problems presenting in general practice, and these have been summarized by Lamberts (1979). While the estimates have varied depending on the sample taken and the country of origin of the survey, typically around 10 per cent of a practice's population can be expected to present with psychological problems (Royal College of General Practitioners et al., 1974). There is thus potentially a very considerable contribution for clinical psychologists to make to primary health care.

Just as the general practitioner needs to be a generalist, rather than a specialist, in medicine, so the clinical psychologist working in the primary care field needs to be a generalist. Patients of all ages are referred, presenting with a wide range of psychological syndromes. To be effective in this varied environment, the psychologist needs to be flexible, and to have at his disposal a variety of skills. He needs to be able to function as a non-directive counselor when appropriate, and he needs specific therapeutic techniques, such as relaxation training, the various biofeedback methods, and techniques of behavior therapy.

I have for three years provided this kind of service to two group practices in Sheffield serving between them a population of 22,500. My preferred method of working is to visit each surgery for one session per week to assess and treat patients referred by the doctors. In this way referral through other agencies, such as psychiatrists, is eliminated. Patients can be seen with little or no waiting in surrounding with which they are familiar.

## TREATMENT METHODS

It is often supposed that psychological therapies can be defined and distinguished from one another with relative ease. However, therapists of different theoretical persuasions observing a therapist at work will describe what they see in radically different ways and according to their own premises (Lazarus, 1971). At the same

Table 1. Distribution of Types of Treatment Received by 149 Patients

| Treatment | Patients |
|---|---|
| GSR Biofeedback | 14 |
| Relaxation | 31 |
| Behavior Therapy | 49 |
| Counseling | 55 |

time, treatment rarely comprises a single component. Besides the non-specific effects of any intervention, there is a counseling element in most behavior therapies, and behavioral features of counseling. For this reason, Table 1, which shows the distribution of different types of treatment received by 149 patients, must be viewed with some caution, since the categories are not necessarily mutually exclusive. It shows roughly that one-third of the patients received treatment which was predominantly physical, that is either relaxation or GSR Biofeedback. The remainder fall into two groups, again roughly equal, one receiving behavioral treatment other than relaxation such as social skills training, response prevention in obsessionals, and enuresis control, whilst the other group was treated by verbal methods only.

## RESULTS

A total of 238 patients, 88 male, 150 female, were seen during the first twenty-six months of the project. A total of 185 were accepted for treatment. An outcome study of 149 patients discharged by October, 1978, has been published (Ives, 1979), showing favorable results.

In an attempt to assess outcome, a global rating of improvement yielded a figure of 72 per cent making a satisfactory progress, more than half to the extent of being symptom free. Such an assessment,

Table 2. Comparison of Doctor/Patient Contacts and Number of Prescriptions Issued for Psychotropic Drugs Between Periods of 3 Months Each, Before and After Treatment.*

| | 3 MONTHS BEFORE | 3 MONTHS AFTER | CHANGE |
|---|---|---|---|
| TOTAL VISITS | 385 | 246 | 36%** |
| TOTAL PRESCRIPTIONS | 205 | 102 | 50%** |

*Numbers indicate totals of 109 patients for whom 3-month follow-up data were available.

**$p<0.00001$, 2-tailed Wilcoxon test.

From Ives, "Psychological Treatment in General Practice," Journal of the Royal College of General Practice, June, 1979, page 346. Reprinted with permission.

Table 3. Comparison of Doctor/Patient Contacts and Number of Prescriptions Issued for Psychotropic Drugs Between Periods of 3 Months Each for Patients Whose Progress Was Followed Up.*

| | 3 MONTHS BEFORE | 3 MONTHS AFTER | 12-15 MONTHS AFTER |
|---|---|---|---|
| TOTAL VISITS | 165 | 104 (37%)** | 94 (43%)** |
| TOTAL PRESCRIPTIONS | 81 | 39 (52%)** | 45 (44%)** |

*Numbers indicate totals of 49 patients for whom 1-year follow-up data were available. Changes from baseline (3 months before) are in parentheses.

**$p<0.002$, 2-tailed Wilcoxon test.

From Ives, "Psychological Treatment in General Practice," Journal of the Royal College of General Practice, June, 1979, page 346. Reprinted with permission.

however, made by myself in retrospect, must be viewed with a good measure of suspicion. A more objective and unbiased record is to be found in the patients' exchanges with their general practitioners--the number of visits made to the surgery, and the number of prescriptions issued for psychotropic drugs. These two variables are measured for the three months immediately prior to referral and for the three months immediately after discharge. Where possible, the same measures were taken for the three month period 12 to 15 months after discharge. Tables 2 and 3 summarize these results.

These results were obtained with relatively short treatment time. The average duration of therapy, excluding patients seen for assessment only, was five half-hour sessions per patient with a range of two to twenty sessions. Seventy per cent required five sessions or fewer. Age range was two to seventy-one years with a mean of 34 years with 22 patients under 16 years of age.

## DISCUSSION

These results support the hypothesis that psychological treatments, to which tension control methods make a very significant contribution, are of value in the primary health care setting. A large number of patients can receive effective treatment in a relatively short time, thus making good use of a scarce resource. At the time of writing, there are only about 500 clinical psychologists in the National Health Service.

Because the techniques of tension control are so useful, it may seem odd to mention a caveat regarding their use. Yet this must be so, since the practitioner of any effective psychological technique must be sensitive to the context in which he uses it. We must be careful not to be too symptom-centered. It is not enough to apply technique alone when a person's distress arises from, for example, marital problems, intolerable housing conditions or dehumanizing employment. Simply to apply technique in such cases is no different from the routine prescription of psychotropic drugs, and does nothing to help the person resolve the difficulties responsible for the appearance of the symptoms. In this context, tension control methods become a vital adjunct to therapy, but not a replacement for the effort to help the patient change, or adapt to, his life situation.

## THE FUTURE

The study described here was uncontrolled, and although there is indirect statistical evidence that spontaneous remission did not play a large part in the results obtained (Ives, 1979), nothing can replace a properly controlled study. I shall shortly be starting a survey lasting four years in which patients receiving psychological treatment will be compared with a matched control group who will receive nothing except the usual treatment from their general practitioner. For a number of reasons, the idea of random allocation of patients to treatment and no-treatment conditions is not possible, thus necessitating very careful matching of the two groups. From a pool of potential control subjects a group will be selected which is matched with respect to age, sex, socio-economic class, problem (type, duration and severity), and background variables including previous doctor/patient contacts, stressful life events, symptom levels and personality variables. In addition, analysis of outcome data will show any significant interactions between variables. The experimental and control groups' initial data can then be examined to check their similarities; if significant differences are detected at this stage, a different control group can then be selected from the original pool including the interaction criteria.

It is hoped that this study will more precisely delineate both the nature and extent of changes induced by exposure to an eclectic psychological treatment.

## REFERENCES

Ives, G., 1979, Psychological treatment in general practice, Jnl. Roy. Col. Gen. Prac., 29:343.

Lamberts, H., 1979, Problem behavior in primary health care, Jnl. Roy. Col. Gen. Prac., 29:331.

Lazarus, A. A., 1971, "Behavior Therapy and Beyond," McGraw-Hill, New York.

Royal College of General Practitioners, Office of Population Census and Surveys, and Department of Health and Social Security, 1974, "Morbidity Statistics from General Practice," second national study, 1970-71.

# RELAXATION TRAINING -- THE MISUNDERSTOOD AND MISUSED THERAPY

Bruce Paul, M.A., M.A.Ps.S.

Carramar Clinic
Parkside, South Australia

SUMMARY

What is relaxation training?

1. A self-control technique that improves with regular practice.

2. Often the core of a therapeutic program, integrated with other self-control measures.

3. Usually most effective when administered "live" by the therapist responsible for the total program.

## Relaxation is Misunderstood and Misused When:

1. It is regarded as an extra that may be of some help when added on to an existing program.

2. It is used routinely without regard for the time and manner of its introduction.

3. There is failure to give the client an understanding of its nature and how it works.

4. There is failure to motivate and assist the client to practice regularly.

5. There is failure to employ methods to facilitate transfer to life situations.

6. There is failure to recognize its many applications.

## RELAXATION

### 1. A Self-control Technique that Improves with Regular Practice

This definition of relaxation comes from Goldfried and Trier (1974). They studied relaxation as an active coping skill and found that "individuals who had been trained in the use of relaxation as a self-control coping skill expressed greater satisfaction with the procedure than those for whom it was construed as more or less a method for passively reducing anxiety".

A feeling of increased control of one's reactions is an interesting outcome of relaxation training. People who have learned to relax and have successfully applied relaxation in their life situations report this feeling of control, and as well a feeling that they have begun to take responsibility for their own lives and their own health. They took a responsible step when they decided to learn to relax. Once they learned that voluntary control of physiological functions was possible they felt more responsible for their reactions to stressful events in their lives. They began to feel actively involved in changing their responses in these situations.

On the other hand, when a person is learning to relax and learning the voluntary control of autonomic functions the situation is rather paradoxical, in the sense that control of these functions is established by the "letting go" of all efforts to control them. Benson (1975) regards the passive, accepting, "let it happen" attitude as the most important component of the relaxation response.

So there is this passive, accepting component in relaxation training, but when facing the challenges and stresses of life one may feel actively involved in employing relaxation as a coping skill. But however we conceptualize relaxation and whatever method we use in the teaching of relaxation, regular practice is essential. Recently I read a book on the application of meditation techniques to stress-related disorders, and a recurring phrase in the book was "conscientious meditators". The author was stating that those who practiced their meditation regularly got the best results.

### 2. Often the Core of a Therapeutic Program, Integrated with other Self-control Measures

Because many of the people who come to us for help are experiencing difficulty controlling their anxiety, or complain that they are not really enjoying life because they are so tense, or present with stress-related disorders, frequently relaxation training will be the core of the therapeutic program. Sometimes it is appropriate to introduce other methods of self-control into the program, for example, desensitization, rational thinking and assertive training.

I find that often the sequence in therapy is something like this: after spending time getting to know the patient and giving him the opportunity to get to know me, I introduce relaxation training. I explain its nature and how it can help the client cope with his specific problems. Then a few sessions may be devoted to teaching the skill and helping the client begin to apply it to his life situations. A cassette recording of the relaxation instructions may or may not be used, depending on the individual client.

The sources of excessive tension in a client's life are more clearly identified, and of course frequently these are associated with habitual ways of viewing himself or reacting to others. Then desentization or rational thinking or assertive training may be introduced. It is important for the client to discover for himself that once he achieves a degree of relaxation in the tension areas of his life, it is easier for him to think rationally and act confidently in these situations that have been troubling him.

3. Usually most Effective when Administered "Live" by the Therapist Responsible for the Total Program

Outcome in therapy is always influenced by the therapist-client relationship. There is a new client, he is rather tense and perhaps apprehensive about seeking help. His initial need is sensitive and patient listening. He is responsive to a counselor who is natural and warm and prepared to listen rather than talk. A relationship of this kind facilitates the expression of feelings and the release of tension, and in this context it seems natural and appropriate for the therapist to introduce relaxation.

In my view, this introduction should be a "live" administration of the relaxation procedure by the therapist. There are three reasons for this. First, client response is enhanced because relaxation has become part of the ongoing therapist-client relationship. Second, the therapist's observations of the client's response make possible appropriate modifications to the procedure. Third, because the therapist has administered relaxation "live" and observed the client's reactions, there is a better integration of the procedure into the total therapeutic program.

## RELAXATION MISUNDERSTOOD AND MISUSED

1. It is Regarded as an Extra that may be of Some Help when Added on to an Existing Program

It may be of some help when used in this way, but I have found that relaxation training is most effective when it is an integral part of a program, and, as I have indicated, often it is the central therapeutic procedure of a program.

When relaxation is regarded as an extra, an adjunct to therapy, we can find ourselves in the situation where someone will approach us and ask, "Would you mind giving this person some relaxation, and I will be continuing with my psychotherapy?". Here there is a failure to integrate relaxation with counselling or psychotherapy, and possibly a failure to appreciate the difficulties that can arise when two therapists are concurrently seeing the same person.

## 2. It is Used Routinely without Regard for the Time and Manner of its Introduction

While relaxation training may be appropriate for nearly all clients who are experiencing excessive tension, when it is introduced and how it is introduced will be different for each client. It may be introduced in the first session or its introduction may be delayed until the third or fourth session. When relaxing a person for the first time the procedure may be brief, just a few minutes, or it may be longer. The rationale that is given may be brief and simple, or it may involve a longer discussion. A cassette recording of the relaxation instructions may or may not be used in the training program.

A routine use of relaxation that I consider to be inappropriate is the handing out of cassettes to clients who complain of anxiety. Recently a woman was referred to me for the treatment of distressing panic reactions. I discovered that four months previously she had been admitted to hospital in a state of panic, where she was investigated medically and then referred to someone who counselled her and handed her a relaxation cassette. She had little understanding of the nature of relaxation and how it might help her and after listening to the cassette a couple of times she put it aside. Her anxiety and feelings of panic and loss of control returned. We talked together about the stresses in her life, her panic reactions, and intervention with relaxation training. I relaxed her and she decided to practice the relaxation exercise at home without the aid of a cassette. When I saw her a week later, she decided to take the cassette. She began listening to the cassette regularly, we talked about the application of the relaxation technique to her life situations, and gradually she is learning to control her anxiety.

## 3. There is Failure to Give the Client and Understanding of its Nature and how it Works

I have found it is important to give clients some understanding of the nature of anxiety, some understanding of its physiological and psychological components, and then go on to indicate how relaxation training can bring about changes in both areas. With relaxation training there is a lowering of tension level and a slowing down of bodily processes, and this feeling of physical relaxation often facilitates cognitive changes. Frequently the change in thinking is in the direction of a more accepting and less demanding attitude towards oneself and towards others.

There are many facets of relaxation training that are gradually experienced by clients, and I have found it is helpful to explore and seek to understand these experiences in a counselling relationship.

## 4. There is Failure to Motivate and Assist the Client to Practice Regularly

Some people respond quickly to relaxation training and report immediate benefit, although in the third or fourth week they may feel discouraged because they are not doing so well. For others the response is gradual over a longer period of time. So therapists have to be patient and do all they can to motivate clients to practice regularly.

Sometimes it takes a client several weeks to reach the stage of acceptance of relaxation training and the discipline of daily practice. I have seen clients with a high anxiety level that has been with them most of their lives and who are forever complaining about it respond to relaxation training after regular practice over a period of several months. Some clients who have been relaxing regularly for years report the long-term benefits, and it seems to be their intention to go on relaxing for the rest of their lives.

## 5. There is Failure to Employ Methods to Facilitate Transfer to Life Situations

Relaxation training is incomplete if a client learns to relax when he is with the therapist and when he is in a quiet room at home, but doesn't learn how to transfer methods of relaxation and self-control to the tension areas of his life.

There are numerous things we can do to bring about this transfer. I have found that once a person has learned to relax and has become familiar with the relaxation technique through regular practice, it is helpful to relax and loosen up for just a few seconds many times during the day, whenever he thinks of it. One way he can do this is to repeat quietly to himself a sentence from the relaxation exercise, which then becomes a cue for relaxation. I have already indicated that with some clients it is appropriate to introduce desensitization or rational thinking or assertive training to help bring about the desired relaxation and confidence in situations in which tension is being experienced.

6. There is Failure to Recognize its Many Applications

If we are working in this area it is sometimes important to state that we are not advocating a complete absence of stress and tension. A life without stress and challenge would be no life at all. In some situations we function better when there is some tension. Our concern is to offer help to people who are experiencing excessive tension, often the result of prolonged, unremitting stress over many years. People in their teens or twenties may be reacting to stress with worry and tension that slowly accumulates and results in a stress-disorder in their forties or fifties. Relaxation training then, can be viewed not only as a method of treatment for the consequences of excessive tension in the middle-aged, but also as a preventive measure for younger age groups.

Let me now mention some of the applications of relaxation training. It is a method of treatment for high levels of anxiety and the concomitants of anxiety such as tension headaches and insomnia, for phobic reactions, for medical conditions that are generally regarded as stress-related disorders, (for example, cardiovascular and respiratory disorders), and for unwanted behaviors that occur mainly when there is a high tension level (for example, aggression and exhibitionism). A man was referred to me because he was frequently exposing himself to girls. Relaxation training over several months reduced his tension level and gave him control over this behavior. It is also a treatment for family tensions and conflicts. Relaxation training can bring about a reduction of husband-wife and parent-child tensions. The mother of a retarded boy responded well to relaxation training, and the outcome was a calmer approach to difficulties in the home and some changes in the boy's behavior. Relaxation can also help alcohol, drug addiction and sexual dysfunction.

Group relaxation training has some advantages over individual training. At the weekly sessions, in addition to relaxation training, time is devoted to group discussion, giving trainees the opportunity to report benefits derived from the training or request help with difficulties being experienced. These discussions can be very stimulating, frequently focusing on problems associated with lifestyle and the pressures of daily living. I see the group approach as a preventive measure for members of the general public who are getting along reasonably well in their lives and occupations, but who experience inappropriate tension and want to do something about it.

So relaxation training has these applications. We find that people are learning to relax, and learning to approach life with renewed interest and confidence. Then I ask myself, "Is this enough?" I ask this question because I sense that many of the people I am seeing are troubled by a feeling that their lives are rather empty and devoid of meaning. I am finding in myself a growing interest in exploring the limits in this area of relaxation and meditation. I am finding it important to lose the sense of rush and make space for silence in my life.

Pelletier (1977), a clinical psychologist, has suggested that some of the methods of relaxation and meditation that are being practiced can be the beginning of a personal quest for deeper meanings in everyday experience. This quote from Pelletier gives some idea of his emphasis: "Living each moment as clearly and fully as possible allows the individual to know which step or direction is next in his life path. Being able to tolerate the ambiguity of not programming an entire life, nor following a preconceived pattern, but remaining open to innovation and insight, is the essential challenge."

So I am finding that relaxation training can be an absorbing challenge for both therapist and client.

## REFERENCES


Benson, H., 1975, "The Relaxation Response," William Morrow, New York.

Goldfried, M. R. and Trier, C. S., 1974, Effectiveness of relaxation as an active coping skill, Journ. of Abn. Psy., 83:348.

Pelletier, K. R., 1977, "Mind as Healer, Mind as Slayer," Dell, New York.

# HOW CHILDREN LEARN THE SKILL OF TENSION CONTROL

A. B. Frederick, Ph.D.

Professor of Physical Education
State University of New York
Brockport, New York

Children should learn to relax for the same reason they learn the skills of reading, writing and arithmetic. Tension control is a basic skill. Is such a skill worthy of "Fourth R" status in the curriculum of basic education? Is it indeed presumptious to claim that something called "relaxation," essentially a non-verbal skill, should be equated with the "Three Rs," the latter forming the essential verbal and symbolic foundation for literacy and technology? I believe the answer to such questions to be in the affirmative (Frederick, 1979).

There is no question about the relationship between tension-related disease and health (Jacobson, 1970; Selye, 1976). Individuals who are skilled at relaxation are less likely to become the victims of tension and stress. Tension control training is primarily conceived as an important aspect of preventative medicine. But beyond disease prevention, learning to relax provides the child with a wonderful introduction to the human organism and its possibilities when viewed as an instrument to be self-run. This is the basis of the "inner curriculum" (Gallwey, 1976).

Tension is always a function of the voluntary musculature. When we exert any effort inclusive of thinking, (Malcolm, 1978; Jacobson, 1973a), the muscles are involved, contracting in unique and measurable patterns. The technique of muscle relaxation, as contrasted with our general notion of "taking it easy," is psychomotor skill. Once mastered, tension signals from the proprioceptive (inner) environment are easily recognized. The application of such learning is the reduction of inappropriate muscular contraction associated with misplaced efforts of all kinds. Since muscular tension can have a dramatic effect on health, the early acquisition of relaxation strategies in the general education of children should have the effect of reducing the incidence of tension-related disorders in adulthood.

Unfortunately, there exist only meager data to support such a contention. Singer's review of developmental factors and their influence on skill learning (Singer, 1968) and Scott's statement that "organization hampers reorganization" (Scott, 1962) support in general the present view that an early acquisition of the technical skill of relaxation creates the potential for ridding oneself of excessive muscular efforts (bracing) later in life. The cultivated habit of selective relaxation thus tends to replace the more primitive, habitual bracing response of modern, civilized living with new habit patterns.

The discovery that neuromuscular relaxation is a motor skill and is learned and practiced in much the same way as other skilled behavior, was first noted in this century by a persistent scientist named Edmund Jacobson. His early experiments on the startle response, measuring the experimental reaction to a sudden, loud noise (Jacobson, 1926), required that some of his subjects sit as quietly as possible. These investigations led him to study and measure the relaxed state in depth. He developed the method and technique he called progressive relaxation and as a physician he often taught his patients to relax. His methods for instructing individual patients is carefully worked out in his classic medical text, _Progressive Relaxation_ (Jacobson, 1929). Later, he encouraged educators to apply the techniques he developed for purposes of group instruction and was instrumental in training Naval officers in his methods for group training at U.S. Navy air schools (Neufeld, 1951).

Progressive relaxation was first adapted for group instruction by Arthur Steinhaus and Jeanne Norris at the George Williams College in Chicago. Their adaptations of progressive relaxation for college students were validated in a study supported by the U.S. Office of Education (Steinhaus and Norris, 1964). Following the lead of Steinhaus and Norris, a Chicago physical educator, Cosmo Cosentino, assisted by Bernardine Lufkin, director of education for the Foundation for Scientific Relaxation began an extensive action research project in the Chicago Heights elementary schools with certain aspects having been pilot tested earlier at Beloit College (Jacobson and Lufkin, 1966). Lufkin's final report (1968) indicated the following results:

1. Methods should be adjusted to meet the varying capabilities of children.
2. Economic background seemed to be a factor in learning.
3. Periodic practice sessions of short duration but over the entire elementary school experience of the child

were recommended.

4. Teachers in the project continued to teach relaxation techniques after the project was officially completed. They had been convinced of the value of such training.
5. It was concluded that the school program in tension control must have the cooperation and support of all school personnel in order to be successful.

During the 1960's my own elementary school physical education classes were introduced to relaxation techniques. In addition to the methodology employed in the Chicago Heights Project, I introduced the elements of various dialogues which were an important feature of a newer, heuristic method of presentation (Frederick, 1967). Children were challenged with such questions as, "What makes your arm go up?" or "Can you show me a 'nothing' face?" As Jacobson had discovered some years earlier (Jacobson, 1973b), children enjoyed the challenge of "running themselves."

Two general methods of teaching tension control to children may be identified. Both methodologies are successfully combined by experienced teachers depending upon class member characteristics and experience. The first is identified as the Deterministic/Analytic Method which adapts the methods of Jacobson in a highly structured series of classes. Such a method has been outlined by Marshall and Beach (1976). The second method which is hueristic in nature and capitalizes on certain features of the process of learning. It might be described in general terms as the Method of Guided Discovery. Since less information is available on the themes of instruction associated with the latter methodology, I have elected to concentrate upon such themes in the present paper.

Teaching relaxation techniques to children from the point-of-view of guided discovery focuses upon the learning process. Thematic guidelines may be described as follows:

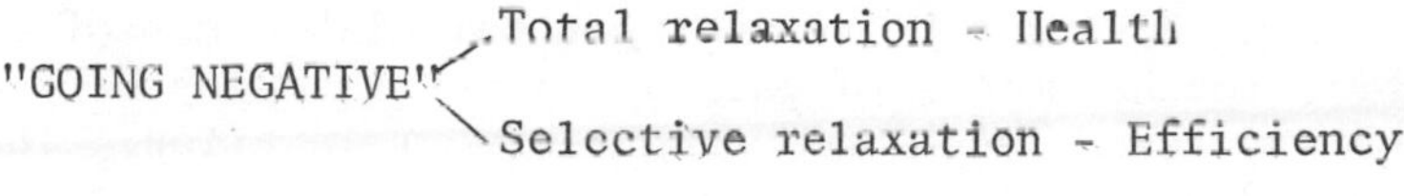


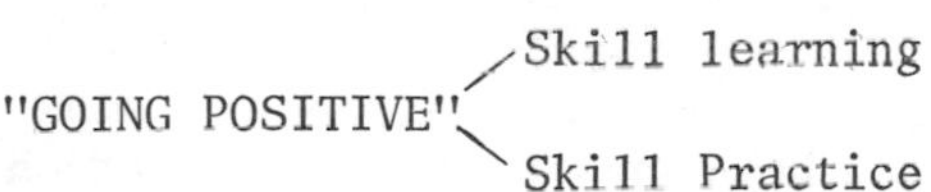


"Going negative" simply refers to the temporal aspect of the relaxed state. The task is either to achieve complete rest or to selectively relax those muscles which are not involved in the performance of tasks associated with one's daily routine. The ability to "go negative" can be tested with electromyographic (EMG) apparatus. The EMG measures the microvoltage present in the neuromuscular system from moment to moment. A person trained to totally relax the musculature would show a gradual progression towards zero microvolts produced when connected to such apparatus. The EMG was employed in the validation strategy of Steinhaus and Norris (1964).

An individual who has learned to relax thoroughly will have gained a working concept of rest that matches the physician's instruction to "take it easy." Individuals who can relax in this sense are subject to fewer tension-related disorders. Observing children at rest often reveals a certain few who should be given training beyond that suggested here for general education. It is also important that children learn how to observe themselves and others at rest. In most cases, I have found that children are able to develop good observational skills.

Going negative can also be a selective process. This means that the individual should be able to move more efficiently as a result of training. Movement education has become an important curricular feature of elementary school physical education. Such programs can easily accommodate tension control methodology. Indeed, the physical education of children is seriously deficient when relaxation is completely ignored. In calling for a new image for physical education, Steinhaus (1963) refers to the "the full activity spectrum" meaning that "going negative" or "zero activity" is the compliment of the more common exercise/activity program.

"Going negative" can be differentially applied. This means very simply that one should use only those muscular efforts that are necessary to accomplish a specific task efficiently. All too often, relaxation is equated only with rest. Laban (1963), whose theories form the foundation of movement education, has pointed out the differences as well as the complimentary nature of effort and relaxation in movement.

"Going positive," indicating a calculated use of tension, is central to the method of guided discovery employed by a majority of those who teach Jacobson's progressive relaxation. The use of brief efforts during relaxation training must be explained since such a technique seems to run counter to the objectives of tension control. Jacobson (1978) states quite properly that "an effort to relax is always failure to relax." He has frequently repeated this point to illustrate the difference between technical relaxation and relaxation inferred by programs requiring concentration, the repetition of phrases or sounds, other imaginative activity or autosuggestive methods to produce a "relaxed state." A person who has been trained to relax in the technical, Jacobsonian sense simply "goes negative" to achieve either rest or selective muscle tension reduction without the need for any special preparatory effort.

"Going positive" is my own elaboration of special features of the training procedure per se. It refers specifically to the pedagogy of tension control. Minimal effort in the form of brief and slight contractions of specific muscle groups are commonly employed in instruction. Once induced, such tension is used to train the learner in self-observation. If tension is to be recognized, it must first be produced. The recognition process proceeds with progressively decreasing tension induction.

To better understand the pedagogical technique I call "going positive," imagine a learner practicing self-observation while seated in a comfortable chair with padded arms. The learner raises the forearm of the left upper limb as illustrated in Figure 1. While it is raised, the learner attempts to identify specific signals of tension arising from the muscle groups involved. During such practice, the learner may report one of three types of observations:

1. The learner is unable to discriminate between muscle groups which are active and those which are, in general, at rest. Such an inability to report sensations arising directly from the central regions of the primary contracting muscle (the biceps), indicated by the shaded area in Figure 1, is common among beginning students.

2. The learner may report sensations of stretch or strain located near the joint (in the present example near the elbow). Stretching skin is also sometimes mistaken for the elusive signal from the muscle proper.

3. The learner accurately reports the sensation of contraction arising in the biceps muscle (shaded region in Figure 1). Jacobson calls such an ability the discrimination of the "Bell sense" (attributed to Sir Charles Bell who was the first to suggest that the muscles possessed a sensory function sometimes referred to as

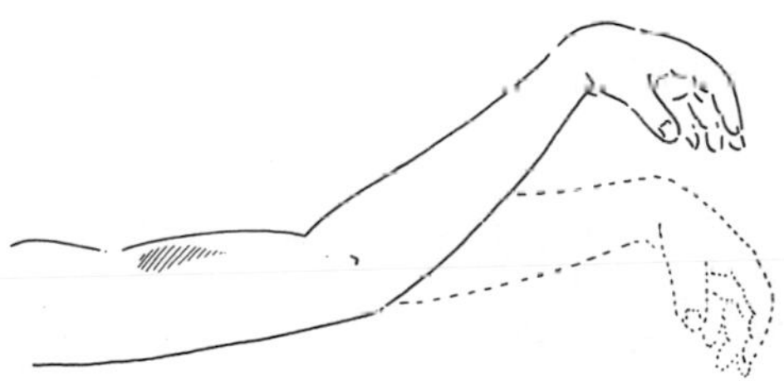

Fig. 1 "Going positive" with the elbow flexors.

"muscle sense"). When accurate observations are forthcoming, the learner is encouraged to attempt to identify the presence of contraction when less tension is induced for example, by only slightly raising the forearm (see dotted illustration in Figure 1). Finally, the learner may be asked simply to imagine lifting the forearm to further test the observation of the signal in the presence of only a miniscule contraction of the biceps. The presence of such contractions during imagined movements was shown conclusively by Jacobson a half century ago (Jacobson, 1930).

"Going positive" also has implications for skill learning associated with the normal spectrum of activity in sport and physical education. The learner might be encouraged to contract certain muscle groups isometrically in preparation for the performance of a new movement with novel characteristics. For example, I have employed such techniques rather effectively during gymnastic training sessions. This procedure is mentioned only in passing since it is not specifically related to relaxation instruction per se but might well be considered in the full range of experience in tension control. It would seem therefore that basic training in tension control techniques inclusive of relaxation should have a positive effect on athletic performance.

## GUIDED DISCOVERY: A DIALOGUE WITH FOURTH GRADERS

I have selected one example of the type of dialogue that typifies the method of guided discovery in the introduction of tension control techniques to children. The objective of the interaction which follows was to have children discover some information about "doing nothing" (going negative):

1. To understand that there are bodily functions that we control directly while others are not.

2. To learn that "doing nothing" is not as simple to do as one might believe.

The children (S) participating in taped sessions were fourth graders. The teacher (T) conducting the lesson was the writer. The class was based upon six years of experience teaching children tension control techniques inclusive of those adapted directly from Jacobson's progressive relaxation (Jacobson, 1938), class notes and tape recorded sessions with children. The following dialogue is extracted from one of several introductory lessons one might use with children in Grades 4 to 6.

T - "Today we will have a brief lesson on 'how to do nothing'."

S - Laughter.

T - "Is it possible to do nothing?"

S - Negative responses; e.g. "You'd be dead!"

Note: The array of responses at this point gets some response from most children. They are quick to point out that the heart must beat, the blood flows, eyes blink and we breathe. Occasionally, children mention that the brain is always "thinking" or like comment, which can be dealt with during this dialogue or another which follows.

T - "Can you make your heart stop beating?"

S - After some discussion including imaginative ideas about self-inflicted wounds which are rejected... "No."

T - "Can you stop breathing for an hour?"

S - "No." (Some of the children will know about the world's record, however - twelve minutes approximately.)

T - "Are there other things you must do in order to stay alive?"

S - "You have to think." (In this particular dialogue the thinking theme is followed but I would ordinarily not introduce this independently.)

T - "Do you have to think?"

S - Mixed responses...e.g. "When you're trying to stop thinking you're still thinking about not thinking." (Later on the word "trying" will be associated with other action words indicating "doing.")

T - (At this point, the teacher displays a relaxed face for the students. The eyes have a unfocused appearance, the jaw is relatively limp, and no emotion or attitude is displayed. Jacobson uses his own face as an example in "Progressive Relaxation," Second Edition, 1938, p.93) "Please look at my face."

S - Laughter. (This has always been the first response.)

T - "Was I thinking?"

S - "Maybe." (Other mixed responses.)

T - "Look again very carefully."

S - Children follow directions with less laughter.

T - "Was I thinking?"

S - "No." (But accompanying remarks reveal that children are not confident about their answer.)

T - "What would you have seen if I were thinking?"

S - Children indicate uncertainty.

T - Teacher then displays a number of facial expressions for the children to identify. "What about this?" etc.

S - Children identify such things as fear, eye movements, happiness, inner speech etc.

T - (Displaying relaxed face once again) "Look at my face."

S - Children observe carefully.

T - "Was I thinking?"

S - "We couldn't tell." (This is probably the best answer. The children may believe that thinking is occurring but they do not detect it by observation.)

T - "Then it is possible to stop doing those things that provide others with clues about our thoughts?"

S - "Yes."

T - "What did my face tell you when it was relaxed?"

S - "Nothing." (This response is often accompanied with insightful statements about "doing nothing.")

T - "Can you make a 'nothing' face?"

S - Children are given some time to replicate the teacher's relaxed face but usually cannot control the eyes and very often smile or laugh audibly. Two or three trials follow with approximately the same result.

T - "Why can't you show me a 'nothing' face?"

S - "It's too hard!"

Note that at this point, the teacher will have made good progress towards accomplishing the objectives of the lesson noted on preceding page. There needs to be some follow-up on the difference between autonomic and voluntary functions of the human organism. For example, when told to do something upon hearing a signal, children will perform a variety of movements. They realize that such performances are different from those ongoing functions such as the heart beat which they cannot willfully start or stop.

A dialogue can be designed that will lead them to the discovery that it is their muscles that are primarily responsible for willed movements of all kinds and that the muscles play an active role in thinking as well.

## CONCLUSION

In his novel, "Island," Huxley (1962) provideds an enlightening perspective about the basics of education in a utopian society on the isle of Pala. The Under-Secretary of Palanese Education asks a visitor, "In the organic hierarchy, which takes precedence (in a child's education) - his gut, his muscles or his nervous system?" The reader discovers that the Palanese attempt to educate their children by combining Western, scientific symbolism with the raw, mystical experience of the East; an integration of verbal and non-verbal education.

For more than a decade, American education has wrestled with three sets of educational objectives which are often regarded, in true Western tradition, as mutually exclusive. Called taxonomies of educational objectives, elements from the cognitive, affective and psychomotor domains are examined (Bloom, 1956, Krathwohl, 1964 and Harrow, 1972). Because of tradition and the need to develop adequate tests of intellectual abilities and skills, the cognitive domain ("nervous system," symbolism, the "Three Rs" etc.) is given preeminence. The affective domain ("gut," organic system, emotion etc.) is given lip service and the psychomotor domain ("muscle," exercise, physical education etc.) is often neglected altogether.

Although a "Fourth R" (relaxation) has been proposed in this paper which could result in the development of the very useful and desirable goals of tension reduction and tension control, there is the more important consideration of the development of an integrated taxonomy of educational objectives. Such a taxonomy would focus our attention on the interrelationships of "gut, muscle and nerve." The "action pattern" domain suggested by Loree (1965) and the conclusions about the dominance of our "presumptious brain" forwarded by Simeons (1962) would strongly favor a "Fourth R" for education.

As we examine the "Fourth R" in this latter sense, it is

apparent that our "nervous education" is at least part responsible for our "nervous society." A tension control program in this, more universal sense would help to balance the emphasis on "nerves" by granting appropriate time in the curriculum for "gut" and "muscle."

REFERENCES


Bloom, Benjamin S., ed., "Taxonomy of Educational Objectives Handbook I: Cognitive Domain", David McKay Co., New York (1956).

Frederick, A. B., 1967, Tension control in the physical education classroom, Jnl. of Health, Phys. Edu. and Rec., 10:42.

Frederick, A. B., 1979, Relaxation: Education's Fourth "R". ERIC Clearinghouse on Teacher Education, Washington, D. C.

Gallwey, W. T., 1976, "Inner Tennis," Random House, New York.

Harrow, A. J., 1972, "A Taxonomy of the Psychomotor Domain," David McKay Co., New York.

Huxley, A., 1962, "Island," Harper and Row, New York.

Jacobson, E., 1926, Response to a sudden unexpected stimulus, Jnl. of Exp. Psy., 9:19.

Jacobson, E., 1929, "Progressive Relaxation," University of Chicago Press, Chicago.

Jacobson, E., 1930, Electrical measurements of neuromuscular states during mental activities - I - Imagination of movement involving skeletal muscle, Am. Jnl. of Phys., 91:576.

Jacobson, E., 1938, "Progressive Relaxation," (2nd ed.), University of Chicago Press, Chicago.

Jacobson, E., 1970, "Modern Treatment of Tense Patients," Thomas Publishers, Springfield, Ill.

Jacobson, E., 1973a, Electrophysiology of mental activities and introduction to the psychological process of thinking, in "The Psychophysiology of Thinking," F. J. McGuigan, ed., Academic Press, Inc., New York.

Jacobson, E., 1973b, "Teaching and Learning", National Foundation for Progressive Relaxation, Chicago.

Jacobson, E., 1978, "You Must Relax," (5th ed.), McGraw-Hill, New York.

Jacobson, E., and Lufkin, B., 1966, "Tension Control in Public Schools," (Part 3), Foundation for Scientific Relaxation, Chicago.

Jacobson, E., and Lufkin, B., 1968, "Tension Control in Public Schools," (Part 4), Foundation for Scientific Relaxation, Chicago.

Kratwohl, D., 1964, "Taxonomy of Educational Objectives Handbook II: Affective Domain," David McKay, Co., New York.

Laban, R., 1963, "Modern Educational Dance," (2nd ed. revised by L. Ullmann), Macdonald and Evans, Ltd., London.

Loree, R., 1965, Relationships among three domains of educational objectives, in "Contemporary Issues in Home Economics - A Conference Report," National Education Association, Washington, D. C.

Malcolm, N., 1978, Thinking, Seminar paper for the Center for Philosophic Exchange, State University College at Brockport, Brockport, N.Y.

Marshall, M., and Beach, C., 1976, A method for teaching tension control in the elementary school, in "Proceedings of the Second Meeting of the American Association for the Advancement of Tension Control," F. J. McGuigan, ed., University Publications, Blacksburg, Va.

Neufield, W., 1951, Relaxation methods in U.S. Navy air schools, Am. Jnl. of Psychia., 108:132.

Scott, J. P., 1962, Critical periods in behavioral development, Science, 138:949.

Selye, H., 1976, "The Stress of Life," (2nd ed.), McGraw-Hill, New York.

Simeons, A. T., 1962, "Man's Presumptious Brain," E. P. Dutton, New York.

Singer, R. W., 1968, Motor learning and human performance, in "Developmental Factors and Influence on Skill Learning," The Mcmillan Co., New York.

Steinhaus, A., 1963, "Towards an Understanding of Health and Physical Education," William C. Brown., Dubuque, Iowa.

Steinhaus, A., and Norris, J., 1964, "Teaching Neuromuscular Relaxation," George Williams College, Chicago.

# BEHAVIORAL HEALTH CHANGE THROUGH TENSION CONTROL LEARNING IN ADULT EDUCATION CLASSES

J. Macdonald Wallace, M. Phil., D.P.E., Dip. Ed., F.R.S.H.

Principal Lecturer in Health Education (retired)
West London Institute of Higher Education
Hove, Sussex, England

"Restless, unfixed in principles and place,
In power unpleased, impatient of discrace;
A fiery soul, which, working out its way,
Fretted the pigmy body to decay
And o'er informed the tenement of clay."
John Dryden, "Achitophel"

The author of this paper is an educator and eschews any suggestion of therapeutic treatment in his work.

Learning has been described as the modification of behavior as the result of experience. The intention of the courses described in this paper was to provide the kind of understanding and experience that hopefully might lead to changes in excessive stress behavior that diminished the health of the individual. Any therapeutic benefit that accrues is derived from the change in stress behavior of the individual student and not from the behavior of the tutor.

The courses were started in 1956 in New Zealand when the author, then a lecturer in health and physical education, was invited by the adult education department of Otago University to organize a keep-fit class. Some universitites still have departments of adult education. Others have extra-mural departments. Yet others have opted for a department, school or center of continuing education. Whatever the title, the work is much the same. A publication of the Vancouver adult center in 1973 defined it as follows:

Adult Education is a systematic education in that it involves a sequence of planned purposeful learning experiences under

> the continuing supervision of an education agent. It is peripheral to an adult's primary role in society and it derives its ethos and ethic from the society in which it occurs.

The New Zealand Council for Adult Education, wrestling with new terminology, proposed a definition:

> Continuing Education is the education, both vocational and non-vocational, of those whose main occupational role is no longer that of student.

For various reasons this education may be offered within the university or non-university sectors.

Traditionally, keep-fit classes offer various forms of exercises and a variety of recreational activities which, it is hoped, will improve muscular efficiency and strength and cardiovascular endurance. In the early University of Otago courses, the title "Keep Yourself Fit" was used. The aim of the course, as expressed to prospective students in the brochure was

> ....to help you understand yourself better and to help you react more positively in stress situations to the benefit of your own health.

## STRESS, TENSION AND RELAXATION

The first session covered, in broad terms, the meaning and the effects of stress, tension, and relaxation, and how these may influence the health of the individual.

This tutor's views on these matters have been strongly influenced by the works of Edmund Jacobson (1929, 1948), first encountered in the early 1950's and by the writings and researches of Hans Selye (1956). Each of these distinguished scientists has made a unique and seminal contribution to the health knowledge of mankind. Yet it is one of the scientific curiosities of our time that in the lengthy bibliographies that accompany the prolific publications of each of these brilliant men, whose works relate to each other like the proverbial horse and carriage, the name and works of the other are studiously ignored, just as if he had never existed.

Each course, in the early days, lasted for twelve weeks, the class meeting for two hours once a week. In later years, this was modified to ten weeks. The general plan of the organization of learning experiences was:

1. The student should learn something about the physiological functions of his own body, in relation to stress.

2. He should learn about his own psychological reactions in response to stressors.

3. He should gain some insight into his own interactions with other people, and theirs with him.

4. He should learn about the aging process and the significance of this in the stress reaction.

5. He should learn how to overcome excessive stress through the psychomotor skill that Jacobson called progressive relaxation, and later, tension control.

To achieve this last objective, some twenty or thirty minutes were spent at the end of each meeting learning the techniques of progressive relaxation. It was speculatively assumed by the tutor that as Jacobson had found this to be successful in various therapeutic situations, it might also prove a useful educational tool to help adult students to control their stress reactions. The pattern of the course, throughout the period when measurement took place, is shown in Fig. 1.

## CONTROL OF STRESS

Despite the vast literature, erudite and popular, relating to stress which has been published over the past 25 years, the term is often used in conceptually different and misleading ways even by the experts. The courses described in this paper were based on the biological concept defined by Selye (1956) as

> ....the state manifested by a specific syndrome which consists of all the non-specifically induced changes within a biologic system in response to a stimulus.

For the purpose of the courses, the biologic system has always been the human individual, and the aim of the course, expressed in another way, has always been to help the student understand how he reacts in response to any stressor, and to help him control excessive arousal of "the non-specifically induced changes within (his) biologic system".

It is accepted that this generalized response is not always harmful. Without adequate stress we fail to develop physiologically, psychologically or socially, so many stressors are actively pursued: sailing a boat, climbing a mountain, sexual activity, making an elusive fortune, achieving ephemeral fame. Others we strenuously try

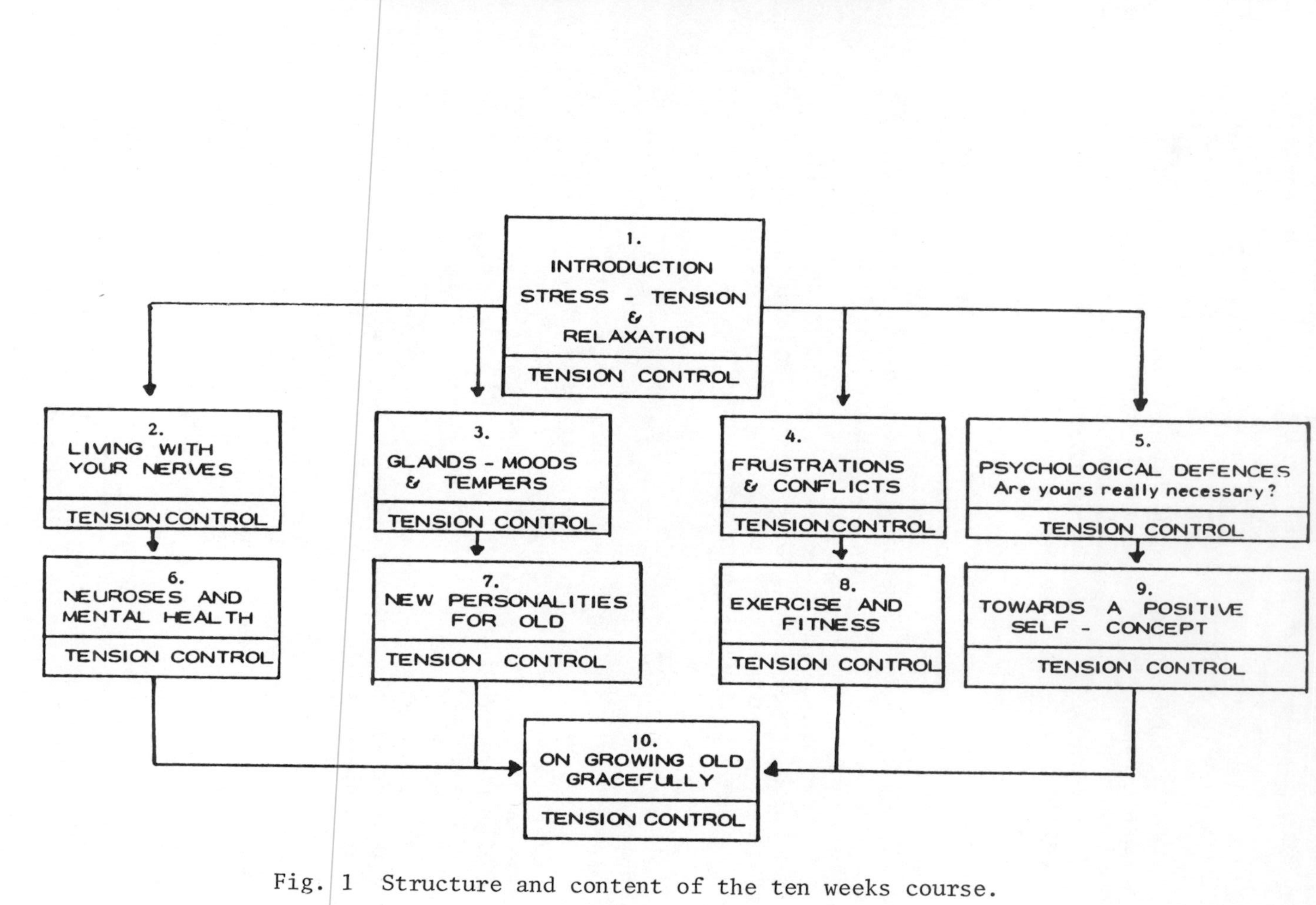


Fig. 1 Structure and content of the ten weeks course.

to avoid. But so complex is the human race that one man's stressor is often another man's joy, and the ability to tolerate stress varies widely from one individual to another.

As Cannon had adequately demonstrated before Selye appeared on the scientific scene, the whole purpose of the physiological arousal that is stress is adaptive. It is the instinctual mobilization for survival purposes of all the resources of the organism to fight a stressor or to flee from a stressor. Each of the myriad physiological changes that take place throughout the body has only one ultimate purpose: to enable the muscles of the body instantly to achieve optimal capacity for contraction for fight or for flight. If neither fight nor flight can be achieved in response to the stressor (and in vast numbers of human situations this is so) then the stress arousal is maladaptive. If the arousal is acute or frequent it may lead to one or more of the so-called stress diseases.

## TENSION CONTROL AND STRESS CONTROL

Although many people throughout history have learned to control this maladaptation through empirical experience, it is to the enduring scientific credit of Edmund Jacobson that, before Cannon or Selye had unravelled the mechanisms of "fight-flight" reaction or "stress", he had demonstrated by ingenious means that

1. When muscle fibers are consciously relaxed "non-specifically induced changes" do not occur in response to a stimulus (stressor) or they are diminished.

2. Where the arousal has already occurred, it can be rapidly reduced through conscious relaxation of muscle fibers.

3. Where a disease of adaptation has already occurred through excessive or chronic arousal but not yet reached an "irreversible" stage of organic change, it may be modified or cured by neuromuscular relaxation. (Jacobson 1920, 1920a, 1927, 1929).

Although nowhere in his voluminous publications does Jacobson refer to biological stress, it is the opinion of this writer that his concept of tension control is the personal key to the control of stress. This point was not clearly grasped when progressive relaxation was introduced into adult education classes some 25 years ago, but it only required the experience of a few groups of students for the author to realize the significance and importance of Jacobson's work in modifying the stress behavior of the individual. In the very first course, and in all subsequent courses, learning the techniques of progressive relaxation was the learning experience that all students stated to be the most important and meaningful for them. It helped them to "...react more positively in stress situations..." It has always been, since 1956, the matrix that integrated the rest of the course.

## MEASURING HEALTH CHANGES

The vast majority of published papers relating to tension control (e.g. Jacobson, 1929, 1964, etc.; McGuigan, 1975, 1976, 1977) or to the control of stress (e.g. Selye, 1976; Levi, 1971; Appley and Trumbull, 1967; Tanner, 1960) are concerned with a therapeutic approach to a specific malady or syndrome: migraine, essential hypertension, cardiovascular disease, peptic ulcers, phobias, insomnia, depression, etc. The therapy has most frequently been conducted on a basis of one patient to one therapist. Occasionally, groups of patients with a common disease have been brought together for clinical or experimental treatment.

With the groups of adult students there were no patients, nor any common health need. Some came with a specific health need which was in most cases unknown to the tutor; others came for professional reasons or from general interest. In the early days no attempt was made to assess entering behavior nor to assess change at the end of the course. The only feedback available to the tutor came from individual reports of some remarkable change in health or in personal relationships in family or job, volunteered by satisfied students at the end of the course or at some later date. It was always accepted as possible that these positive reports arose from cognitive dissonance or from the student's desire to be kind to the tutor, but they were enough to motivate the tutor to continue with the courses for many years in a variety of environments, under the auspices of different universities, local education authorities and other organiazations. The title was changed from "Keep Yourself Fit" to "A Modern Course in Health Education for Adults" (Wallace 1965). This was again changed when, sadly, anything labelled as adult came to mean lascivious, sexy or perverse or all of these things, to "How to Free Yourself from Nervous Tension" (after Gutwirth 1955), which proved to be the most attractive title in the non-university sector. In the more sedate atmosphere of London University classes, the title became "Health Education - Stress and the Individual".

## FINDING A SUITABLE INSTRUMENT

In 1972, the writer returned to New Zealand for a year to lecture in a teachers college. In a small provincial town of some 30,000 inhabitants, including surrounding villages and farms, a series of classes was organized, under the auspices of the local family and marriage guidance council, on the theme "How to Free Yourself from Nervous Tension." The response was good, so it was decided to attempt to measure stress behavior at the beginning and end of the course to find out if any real change took place.

At that time this author knew very little about biofeedback, and, even had he known, had no access to instruments or laboratory facilities. Through the library facilities of Massey University and Palmerston North Teachers College, a number of standardized psychological and personality inventories was examined. These included the Eysenck Personality Inventory, the Minnesota Multiphasic Personality Inventory, the Taylor Manifest Anxiety Scale, the California Psychological Inventory, the Tennessee Self-Concept Scale, the Mood Change Adjective List, and the standard questionnaire used for psychopathological evaluation of patients being admitted to Lake Alice Psychiatric Hospital in New Zealand. Each of these instruments was closely scrutinized to determine its suitability for measuring stress behavior. Each contained pertinent material, some items relating to somatic changes, others to psychological changes, and to changes in self-evaluation or self-concept. All these factors are relevant to stress behavior, but none of the inventories was considered to be adequate for the purpose of the course being organized. It was therefore found necessary to develop a new instrument: the Psychosomatic Tension Relaxation Inventory, PSTRI.

## THE PSTR INVENTORY

The construction of this instrument was based on the assumption that although the instructional objectives of the course were primarily concerned with understanding, and with learning the skill of tension control, it would be in the application of this understanding and of this skill--that is, in adaptive behavior--that any change would be recognized. Moreover, once the understanding and the skill are acquired, the individual student would be the one most likely to recognize changes in himself most accurately. It was therefore considered necessary to develop an inventory relating to forms of stress behavior, or health outcomes arising from stress as commonly described in the literature, and which could be completed in a few minutes.

Stress behavior is much the same as any other behavior, as far as type is concerned. It differs from non-stress behavior quantitatively, qualitatively and chronically, and it is essentially these differences that bring about changes in health patterns of the individual. Any breakdown, or diminution, in health will be associated with physical, mental and social aspects in varying combinations. An inventory which claims to be reasonably vaild as a means of assessing stress behavior would therefore be concerned with items relating to changes in physical, mental and social aspects of health.

In order to find appropriate items, a survey was made of a number of texts relating to stress disorders and psychosomatic disorders.

Eysenck and Eysenck (1963) have argued that the validity of the items of a questionnaire may be supported by the experience views of qualified authorities rather than agreement with an existing criterion. For lack of an existing criterion, it was to experienced authorities that the author looked when devising the PSTR Inventory.

From clinical and experimental studies reported in Appley and Trumbull (1967), Basowitz et al. (1955), Black (1969), Hill et al. (1970), Jacobson (1964), Levi et al. (1971), Maslow (1968), Selye (1956), and Tanner et al. (1960), and from other sources, a fifty item inventory was composed of the kinds of health behavior and experience most commonly reported in the literature. It is on the authority and experience contained in these studies that the inventory claims a reasonable content validity, rather than on the experience of the author.

PSTR INVENTORY

Consider each of the following statements carefully. Decide how it applies to you, then answer by placing your rating in the box opposite the statement, showing the FREQUENCY of the occurence, and the INTENSITY, according to the following scale:-

| | FREQUENCY | INTENSITY | |
|---|---|---|---|
| very often | 4 | 4 | very much |
| often | 3 | 3 | much |
| sometimes | 2 | 2 | some |
| seldom | 1 | 1 | slight |
| never | 0 | 0 | none |

| | FREQ. | INT. |
|---|---|---|
| 1. I suffer from backache.......................... | ...... | ........ |
| 2. My sleep is fitful and disturbed................ | ...... | ........ |
| 3. I get headaches................................. | ...... | ........ |
| 4. My jaws ache.................................... | ...... | ........ |
| 5. I get upset if I have to wait................... | ...... | ........ |
| 6. I am troubled with pains in the back of my neck | ...... | ........ |
| 7. I am more nervous than most other people...... | ...... | ........ |
| 8. I find it hard to get off to sleep............. | ...... | ........ |
| 9. I feel a tightness or tingling in my scalp.... | ...... | ........ |

PSTR INVENTORY (cont.)

| | FREQ. | INT. |
|---|---|---|
| 10. I get stomach trouble........................ | ........ | ..... |
| 11. I lack confidence in myself........................ | ........ | ..... |
| 12. I talk to myself........................ | ........ | ..... |
| 13. I worry about financial problems........................ | ........ | ..... |
| 14. I get embarrassed when meeting people........................ | ........ | ..... |
| 15. I have fears that something dreadful is about to happen........................ | ........ | ..... |
| 16. I get tired during the day........................ | ........ | ..... |
| 17. I get a sore throat in the evening which is not from infection........................ | ........ | ..... |
| 18. I am restless and cannot sit still........................ | ........ | ..... |
| 19. My mouth gets dry........................ | ........ | ..... |
| 20. I have heart trouble........................ | ........ | ..... |
| 21. I feel I'm not much use........................ | ........ | ..... |
| 22. I smoke........................ | ........ | ..... |
| 23. I get "butterflies in the tummy"........................ | ........ | ..... |
| 24. I feel unhappy........................ | ........ | ..... |
| 25. I perspire........................ | ........ | ..... |
| 26. I drink alcohol........................ | ........ | ..... |
| 27. I am self-conscious........................ | ........ | ..... |
| 28. I feel I am going to pieces........................ | ........ | ..... |
| 29. My eyes get tired and sore........................ | ........ | ..... |
| 30. I get cramps in my legs or feet........................ | ........ | ..... |
| 31. My heart pounds rapidly........................ | ........ | ..... |
| Total carried forward | | |

PSTR INVENTORY (Cont.)

| | FREQ. | INT. |
|---|---|---|
| Total carried forward.. | ............ | ......... |
| 32. I am afraid of meeting people.......... | ............ | ......... |
| 33. My hands or feet get cold.......... | ............ | ......... |
| 34. I suffer from constipation.......... | ............ | ......... |
| 35. I take various pills or medicines without doctor's advice.......... | ............ | ......... |
| 36. I find myself in tears rather easily.......... | ............ | ......... |
| 37. I suffer from indigestion.......... | ............ | ......... |
| 38. I bite my nails.......... | ............ | ......... |
| 39. I get a humming in my ears.......... | ............ | ......... |
| 40. I have to empty my bladder.......... | ............ | ......... |
| 41. I have trouble with gastric ulcers.......... | ............ | ......... |
| 42. I get skin troubles.......... | ............ | ......... |
| 43. I get a tightness in my gullet.......... | ............ | ......... |
| 44. I have trouble with duodenal ulcers.......... | ............ | ......... |
| 45. I worry about my job.......... | ............ | ......... |
| 46. I get ulcers in my mouth.......... | ............ | ......... |
| 47. I worry about trivial things.......... | ............ | ......... |
| 48. My breathing is shallow.......... | ............ | ......... |
| 49. I have trouble with ulcerative colitis.......... | ............ | ......... |
| 50. I find it hard to make decisions.......... | ............ | ......... |
| Total Score.... | ............ | ......... |

Name.............................. Age............

Occupation........................ Date...........

Table 1. Mean Scores and S.D. of New Zealand Students

| | Frequency | S.D. | Intensity | S.D. | Mean Age | Age Range |
|---|---|---|---|---|---|---|
| Pre-course | 57.33 | 20.35 | 55.61 | 21.3 | | |
| Post-course | 45.36 | 21.39 | 43.1 | 22.07 | 43.04 | 21-74 |
| Difference | 11.97 | | 12.6 | | | |

Students were asked to complete the inventory at the third meeting of the class, ensuring that late enrollments were involved. A maximum of ten minutes was given for completion.

At the end of the final meeting students were again asked to complete a PSTRI without reference to their previous scoring.

It was hoped from this scoring that it might be possible to find a difference in significance between frequency and intensity, which might give some guidance to understanding the effects of stress. In practice, the correlation between scores in frequency and intensity was so high (.93) that the intensity score was considered redundant and omitted from later experiments.

At the time there was no intention of using the PSTRI as a means of assessing the genral stress status of the individual student, but rather as a means of evaluating a curriculum by finding out if any significant change took place in the mean scores of the experimental population.

## NEW ZEALAND DATA

Forty seven females and 23 males completed the PSTRI in the New Zealand sample. The data are shown in Table 1, and illustrated in Fig. 2.

## ADDITIONAL PRELIMINARY DATA

The following year, in London, 30 more adult students took the course. The data from this group were added to the data of the New Zealand sample. The larger sample of combined groups was made up of 65 females and 35 males, an approximate 2:1 ratio of the sexes which was common to almost all classes enrolled over two decades.

Table 2 shows the mean scores of the combined sample; Fig. 3 illustrates the change graphically.

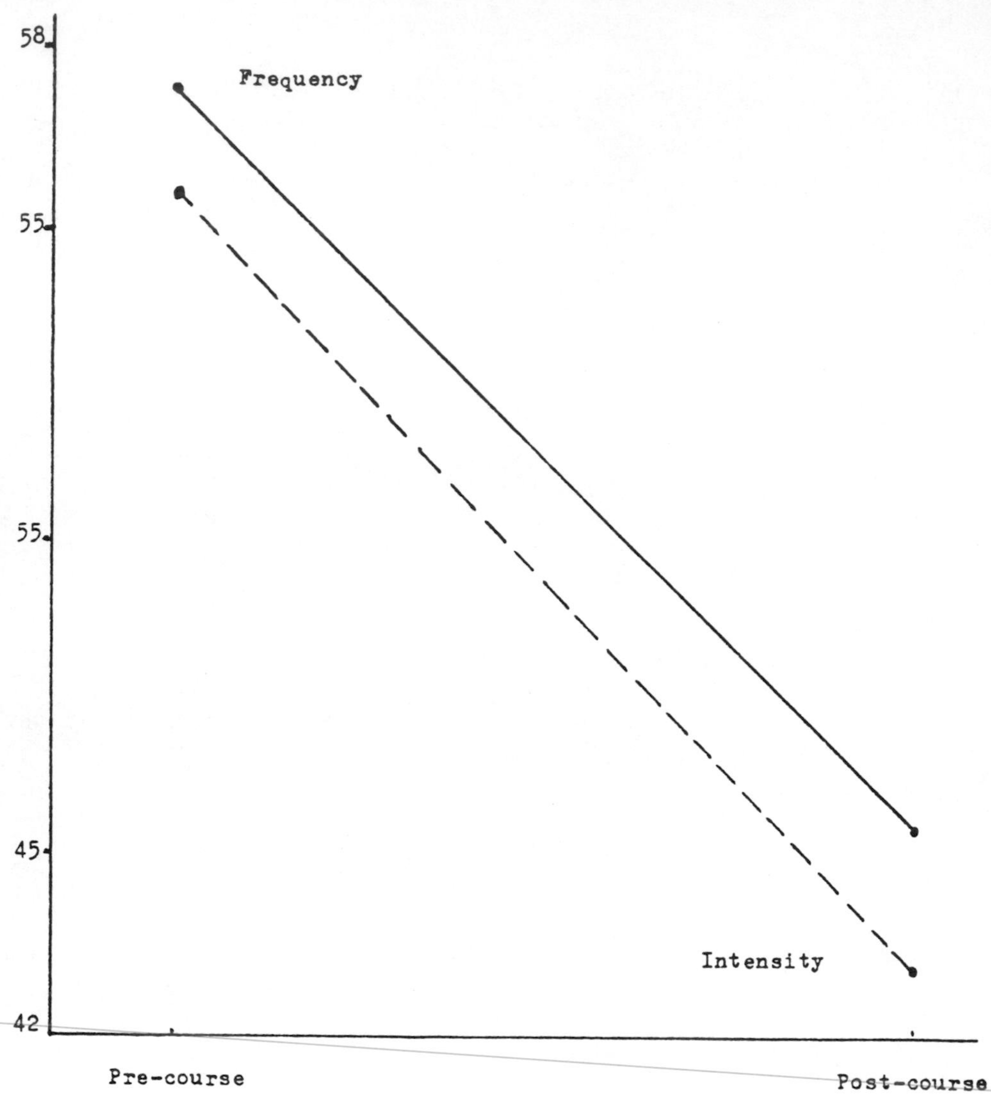


Fig. 2 Mean score change of N.Z. adult students on PSTRI.

Table 2. Mean Scores and S.D. of 100 Students on PSTRI

| | Frequency | S.D. | Intensity | S.D. | Mean Age | | |
|---|---|---|---|---|---|---|---|
| | | | | | all | women | men |
| Pre-course | 58.21 | 21.00 | 57.07 | 21.85 | | 44.7 | |
| Post-course | 46.51 | 21.90 | 44.58 | 22.84 | 45.17 | | 46.03 |
| Difference | 11.70 | | 12.49 | | | | |

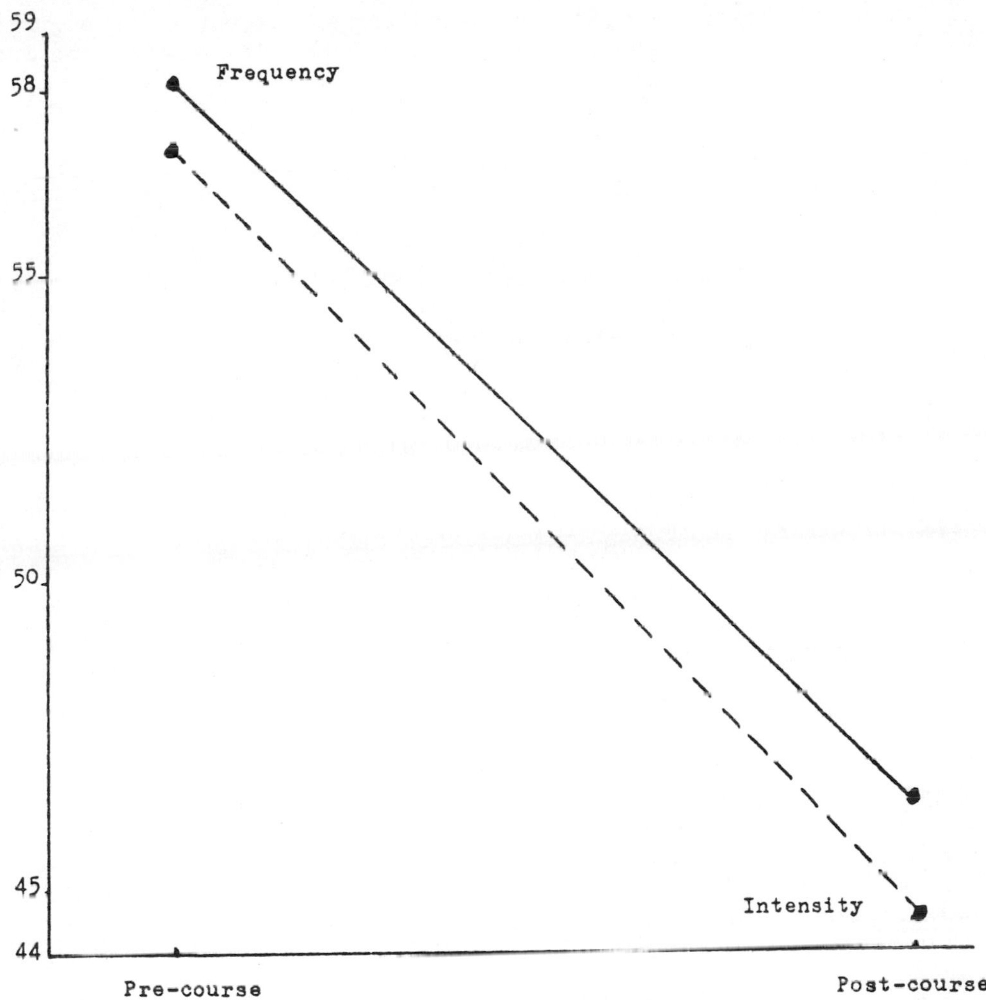


Fig. 3. Mean score change on PSTRI of 100 students in preliminary investigation.

The data of the combined sample was analyzed by computer at the University of London Computing Center by a researcher not connected with the study. In both Frequency and Intensity the change in PSTRI scores of the group was found to be significant at the 0.00001 level. There was no significant correlation between age and PSTRI scores at the beginning or end of the course.

## RELIABILITY OF THE PSTRI

Two hundred and eleven second year college students completed the PSTRI in May 1974. It was intended to re-test in June, but administrative difficulties precluded this, and it was not until the beginning of October that the second PSTRI was completed. The scores were subjected to computer analysis, using the Pearson product-moment formula. A correlation coefficient of .641 was arrived at for test/retest in Frequency, and a coefficient of .644 for test/retest in Intensity. (This was done before the decision was made to discard Intensity as a redundant measure.

This test/retest reliability is not very high, but it must be evaluated in the light of a number of considerations. The nature of the instrument is such that much higher values are not frequently found in practice. Moreover, the time delay between test and retest was much longer than for some other more reliable tests, and this is known to affect the fall-off in reliability.

Later, in the main experimental study, the control group returned, after a ten weeks interval, a reliability coefficient of .77 for frequency scores. Taking into consideration the time interval and the heterogeneity of the adult students the reliability of the PSTRI seems to have reached an acceptable level.

## THE EXPERIMENTAL STUDY

Although the foregoing analyses gave some indication that significant change had taken place in the health behavior of the students taking the course, there still remained the possibility that the change was due to maturation rather than learning through the course. To test this, further courses were set up, and evaluated against a Control group. All subjects in the experimental and control groups were adult students taking part voluntarily in courses offered by the University of London Department of Extra-Mural Studies. This helped to ensure a reasonable degree of socio-economic equivalence.

### The Experimental Group

The Experimental Group was made up of five sub-groups taking the course on Health Education - Stress and the Individual, with the curriculum as already described. Three of the classes lasted for ten weeks (one term) and two lasted for two terms for twenty weeks. All students were self-selected, opting to attend for the satisfaction of some personal need, and all paid a fee to take part in the course. The structure of the course was in Fig. 1, with a similar, but expanded, content for the 20 week course. The distribution is shown in Table 3.

Table 3. Structure of Experimental Group

| Sub-group | Duration (weeks) | N | Females | Males | Mean Age | Age Range |
|---|---|---|---|---|---|---|
| 1 | 10 | 13 | 10 | 3 | 41.85 | 26-56 |
| 2 | 10 | 12 | 6 | 6 | 42.67 | 25-56 |
| 3 | 10 | 20 | 14 | 6 | 41.77 | 24-57 |
| 4 | 20 | 14 | 8 | 6 | 45.73 | 28-60 |
| 5 | 20 | 26 | 16 | 10 | 42.99 | 25-65 |
| Totals | | 85 | 54 | 31 | 42.7 | 24-65 |

The Control Group

The Control Group was made up of 76 adult students attending five different university extra-mural courses in different locations around London. Each control subject completed a first PSTRI, and eight weeks later completed a second PSTRI, without reference to the first. The distribution is shown in Table 4.

Table 4. Structure of Control Group

| Sub-group | N | Females | Males | Mean Age | Age Range |
|---|---|---|---|---|---|
| Transport Engineering | 6 | - | 6 | 27.17 | 24-32 |
| Music | 7 | 5 | 2 | 45.71 | 34-63 |
| Cathedrals of England | 22 | 15 | 7 | 46.77 | 20-71 |
| Geology | 27 | 13 | 14 | 48.59 | 20-71 |
| Archaeology | 14 | 8 | 6 | 38.94 | 20-59 |
| Totals | 76 | 41 | 35 | 44.1 | 20-71 |

None of the students, experimental or control, was aware that an experimental study was being conducted.

The main purpose of the experiment was to see if there would be any significant difference in behavior and attitude between the experimental and control groups as measured by changes in the PSTRI scores. Subsidiary aims were to find out if:

1. A two-term course would produce more significant changes in a group than a one-term course.

2. Changes would take place more significantly in one sex than in the other.

3. Age is a significant variable in determining scores or changes in the PSTRI.

Although 85 experimental subjects completed the pre-course PSTRI, only 75 post-course PSTRI were available at the time of computing the data owing to unavoidable administrative difficulties.

## ANALYSIS OF DATA

The mean values of the PSTRI are shown in Table 5, and indicated the essence of the interaction. This is shown graphically in figure 4.

Table 5. First and Final PSTRI Mean Scores for all Groups

| | | 10 weeks | | | 20 weeks | | | Control | |
|---|---|---|---|---|---|---|---|---|---|
| | N | Mean Score | S.D. | N | Mean Score | S.D. | N | Mean Score | S.D. |
| PSTRI 1 Males | 13 | 56.85 | 18.84 | 15 | 62.67 | 25.30 | 37 | 48.32 | 20.01 |
| Females | 24 | 53.75 | 19.08 | 23 | 62.13 | 24.46 | 39 | 47.31 | 16.62 |
| PSTRI 2 Males | 13 | 47.77 | 19.09 | 15 | 50.33 | 18.05 | 37 | 46.89 | 24.06 |
| Females | 24 | 44.54 | 19.24 | 23 | 50.96 | 22.38 | 39 | 48.87 | 16.93 |
| Mean Change Males | | 9.08 | | | 12.34 | | | 1.43 | |
| Females | | 9.21 | | | 11.17 | | | -1.56 | |
| All | | 9.55 | | | 11.42 | | | -0.11 | |

The raw data were subjected to analysis or variance and analysis of co-variance by computer. Within the limitations of this study, it is possible to draw the following conclusions from these analyses:

1. Participation in the stress reduction courses described led to significant changes in stress-related behavior and to an improvement in health of the experimental group.

2. The changes in stress-related behavior were as significant for a 10 weeks course (.0001) as for a 20 weeks course (.0001).

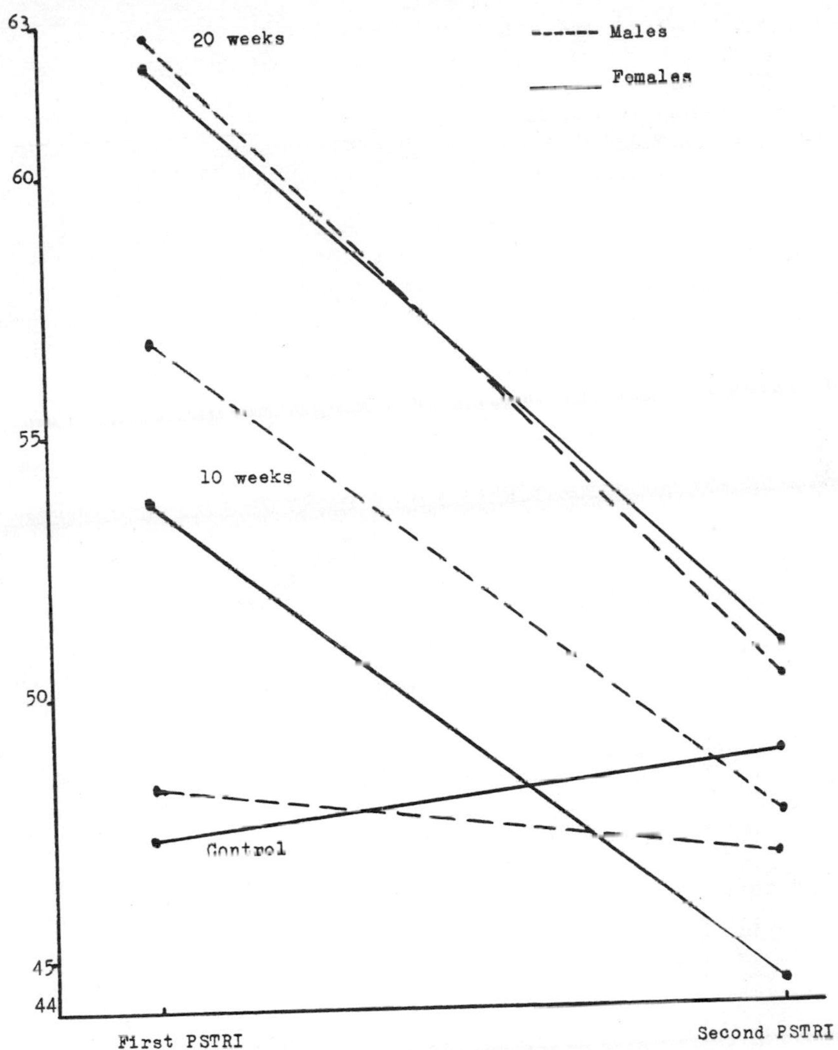


Fig. 4. Changes in PSTRI scores across groups and sexes.

3. The changes in stress-related behavior were not significantly different for men and women students.

4. The changes in stress-related behavior did not vary significantly with age, and were positive at all ages within the experimental group.

5. Change in the control group was practically zero.

RETENTION OF LEARNING

Six months to one year after the end of the experimental courses, 58 subjects returned a third PSTRI. These were matched with the subject's second PSTRI, and the changes analysed by using a t-test for correlated samples. The value of "t" arrived at was 1.059. With 57 degrees of freedom, the critical value of "t" at the .01 level is 2.358. Therefore the Null Hypothesis--that there is no significant difference between scores on the second and third PSTRI--must be retained. So a final conclusion may be drawn.

6. A considerable amount of learning was retained, and the stress reaction of the experimental group was still generally reduced, long after they had completed the course.

The author suggests that there is scope for the development of courses of the kind outlined in this paper within the organization of public adult education classes of many countries, offering an opportunity to learn stress reducing skills to the vast numbers of people who would like to control their own stress, but are not motivated to adopt the role of patient in a therapeutic setting.

## REFERENCES

Appley, M. H., and Trumbull, R., ed., "Psychological Stress: Issues in Research," Appleton-Century-Crofts, New York (1967).

Basowitz, H., 1954, "Anxiety and Stress," McGraw-Hill, New York.

Black, S., 1969, "Mind and Body," William Kimber, London.

Gutwirth, S. W., 1955, "How to Free Yourself from Nervous Tension," Barker, London.

Hill, O. W., ed., "Modern Trends in Psychosomatic Medicine," Butterworths, London (1970).

Jacobson, E., 1920, The use of relaxation in hypertensive states, N.Y., Med. Jnl., 111:419.

Jacobson, E., 1920a, Reduction of nervous irritability and excitement by progressive relaxation. Trans. Sec. Nerv. and Ment. Dis., 53:282.

Jacobson, E., 1927, Spastic esophagus and mucous colitis, Arch. Int. Med., 39:433.

Jacobson, E., 1929, "Progressive Relaxation," University of Chicago Press, Chicago.

Jacobson, E., 1948, "You Must Relax," McGraw-Hill, New York.

Jacobson, E., 1964, "Anxiety and Tension Control," Lippincott, Chicago.

Levi, L., ed., "Society, Stress and Disease," vol. 1., Oxford University Press, London (1971).

Maslow, A. H., 1968, "Towards a Psychology of Being," Van Nostrand, New York.

McGuigan, F. J., ed., "Proceedings of the Second Annual Meeting of the American Association for the Advancement of Tension Control," University Publications, Blacksburg, Va., (1975).

McGuigan, F. J., ed., "Proceedings of the Third Annual Meeting of the American Association for the Advancement of Tension Control," AAATC, Louisville (1976).

McGuigan, F. J., ed., "Proceedings of the Fourth Annual Meeting of the American Association for the Advancement of Tension Control," AAATC, Louisville (1977).

Selye, H., 1956, "The Stress of Life," McGraw-Hill, New York.

Selye, H., 1976, "Stress in Health and Disease," Butterworths, Boston.

Tanner, J. M., ed., "Stress and Psychiatric Disorder," Blackwell, Oxford (1960).

Wallace, J. M., 1965, A modern health education course for adults, Health Ed. Jnl., 24:4.

# RELAXATION TECHNIQUES WITH THE BLIND

Sylvia Dickerson, M.A.

Virginia Rehabilitation Center for the Blind
Richmond, Virginia

## INTRODUCTION

The purpose of this study is to investigate the effectiveness of relaxation procedures as taught to visually impaired adults at the Virginia Rehabilitation Center for the Blind.

The center is a residential facility for visually impaired adults. Trainees come to the center from all parts of Virginia and stay there as long as necessary, depending on the severity of their sight loss.

The objective of the center is to "assist the visually handicapped individual to gain confidence in himself and to achieve the degree of personal, social and/or vocational independence for which he strives." During the day the trainees attend a variety of classes for personal adjustment skills. One of the classes that the center offers is a six-week course in relaxation techniques. This course was initiated by this writer who for six years has dealt with blind trainees on an individual basis as well as in group settings. Experimental work with animals and human subjects shows a severe reaction when sensory input is limited or when subjects are prevented from moving normally (legs tied, small cage, etc.). This research suggests that blindness is a stressful situation in that limiting sensory input and limiting normal movements are two powerful stressors (Bauman and Yoder, 1966).

A common complaint from the trainees, for example, is that they are under physical and emotional stress. The overt form of such complaints is expressed in general anxiety, restlessness, insomnia, fatigue, depression and a variety of psycho-physiological disorders.

Other research, moreover, shows that light deprivation was more stressful than sound deprivation expressed through symptoms of anxiety, difficulty in thinking and concentration. To the extent that this is true, we have a third stressor associated with blindness (Bauman and Yoder, 1966).

Several terms used in this paper need to be defined.

"Rehabilitation Center for the Blind" is a state residential facility which provides comprehensive adjustment services to severely visually impaired individuals. Classes include orientation and mobility, home management skills, recreation, communication skills, and vocational evaluation.

"Trainees" refers to enrolled blind residents at the Rehabilitation Center.

"Visual impairment (visually handicapped, blind)" are used interchangeably in referring to a legally blind individual. A person is said to be "legally blind" if his central visual acuity does not exceed 20/200 in the better eye with correcting lenses or his visual field is less than an angle of 20 degrees. In simpler terms a person is considered "legally blind" if he can see no more at a distance of 20 feet than someone with normal sight can see at a distance of 200 feet. Normal acuity is 20/20; normal field, 180 degrees.

"Stress" and "tension" are used interchangeably as body's response to demands made upon it, be they mentally, emotionally or physically precipitated.

"Relaxation" is any procedure aimed at achieving muscle and mental quietude.

## RELAXATION TECHNIQUES COURSE

Recent literature on relaxation techniques seems to indicate that no advantage has been demonstrated for one method of relaxation training over another, although in some situations a combination of techniques may be more beneficial than either procedure used alone. In most conditions, the simplest training procedure seems to be as effective as the more complex, provided regular practice periods are punctually observed (Taylor, 1978). For this reason, the program at the center is designed to use several techniques throughout the course.

Participants in the course were either self-referred or encouraged by some staff member to enroll in it. The duration of the course was six weeks, with three weekly sessions of at least forty-five minutes each. Because of the visual disability of the participants, the classes were small, the enrollment averaging about four people. The first week was spent discussing various concepts of tension and their effects upon the individual. The following three weeks were planned around practice sessions following "Progressive Relaxation Training" by Bernstein and Borkovec (1973). During the fifth and sixth week, structured and unstructured meditation as described in LeShan's book "How to Meditate" (1974), were added to the sessions. All sessions were instructed by this writer in vivo as against using taped material.

## RESULTS

One objective in planning the course was to make the use of relaxation techniques in coping with stress as beneficial to the trainees when they returned home as it had been during their stay at the center.

Approximately 60 trainees have been enrolled in the relaxation course since it first began in June of 1976. Twenty ex-trainees selected at random were contacted by telephone by a non-instructional staff member who recorded the answers to a follow-up questionnaire which consisted of a self-report of relaxation effectiveness.

The youngest person in the sample was a seventeen-year-old male and the oldest was a seventy-nine-year old female. The education level varied from sixth grade to a masters degree.

The following results were obtained from the contact information:

1. No one in this group had ever had any course or class in any relaxation technique previous to the one offered at the center.

2. Ninety percent of the group were still actively using most of the techniques learned in the course.

3. The reasons given for the continuation of the practice were both physical and psychological. Physical benefits were described as "relaxed muscles," "more daily energy," "falling asleep easily," and "unwinding in the evening." The psychological benefits were "clearer thinking," "improved concentration," "better self-control," and "peace of mind."

4. As to the preferred technique to achieve relaxation, seventy-five percent of the group reported a combination of progressive muscular relaxation in combination with visual imagery. The other twenty-five percent were equally divided between progressive muscular relaxation and visualization as their

technique of choice.

## CONCLUSION

Even though the relaxation course is only one component of a trainee's multimodal rehabilitation program at the center, it appears that the benefits are significant and seemingly of lasting duration.

## REFERENCES

Bauman, M.K., and Yoder, N. M., 1966, "Adjustment to Blindness--Re-Viewed," Charles C. Thomas, Springfield, Ill.

Bernstein, D. A., and Borkovec, T. D., 1973, "Progressive Relaxation Training: A Manual for Helping Professions," Research Press, Champaign, Ill.

LeShan, L., 1974, "How to Meditate," Little, Brown, Boston.

Taylor, C. B., 1978, Relaxation training and related techniques, in: "Behavior Modification: Principles and Clinical Applications," W. S. Agras, ed., 2nd ed., Little, Brown, Boston.

# VOLUNTARY CONTROL OF THE INVOLUNTARY NERVOUS SYSTEM: COMPARISON OF AUTOGENIC TRAINING AND SIDDHA MEDITATION

Malcolm Carruthers, M.D., M.R.C. Path., M.R.C.G.P.
Director, Clinical Laboratory Services
Maudsley Hospital
London, England

Man has spent astronomical amounts of time, energy and money exploring outer space. The search has left him tense, stressful, and at war with himself, his fellow human beings and his surroundings.

At last he is beginning to look inward to the "Last Dark Continent" where the answers to the more basic problems of life are more likely to be found. The scientific approach which enabled him to achieve a considerable degree of control over his surroundings has not led to equivalent mastery of this "inner space". Anatomical mapping, physiological probing and biochemical testing has led to major advances in the treatment of acute illness and some chronic diseases, but we are left with a large number of disorders, particularly in the field of psychiatry and psychosomatic disease, for which modern medical science appears to have no satisfactory solutions.

As Ivan Illich has pointed out in his book "Medical Nemesis" (Illich, 1975) drug-based therapy does not appear to provide the answers, and in some cases the side effects are worse than the disease. There is growing disillusion of the general public and the medical profession alike with both the effectiveness and the desirability of long-term medication. Particularly in alleviating the effects of stress on both mind and body.

Consider some of the drawbacks of tranquilizers for example. These "drug crutches" as they have been called by Professor Malcolm Lader do little to get at the root of the disorders for which they are given, but merely turn off the warning signals. Their usage is particularly under attack in the United States where a congressional Committee investigating drug abuse has reported that 44.6 million prescriptions were made out for Valium last year. World-wide 650,000 tons are consumed annually. Habituation to tranquilizers can occur within a few weeks of their regular usage, they can produce acute rage reactions (Salzman et al., 1974) and increased hostility (Kochansky et al., 1977). Withdrawal syptoms can include both worsening of anxiety symptoms and increased aggressiveness or acute psychotic episodes (Gordon, 1979).

Disturbing evidence has also recently come to light that these compounds may promote growth of various tumors, including breast cancer in experimental animals (Horrobin, 1979). They also impair neuromuscular co-ordination for prolonged periods (Clayton, 1976). It has recently been reported that road traffic accidents are considerably higher in people taking either tranquilizers or sedatives (Skeggs, Richards and Doll, 1979). It is alarming to think of the vast number of people who must be driving cars and operating machinery under the influence of these compounds, particularly as their action is potentiated by alcohol. A recent study showed that 50% of aircrew on long-distance flights, including pilots and navigators, were intermittently taking either tranquilizers or sleeping pills, often only a few hours before their flights (Hawkins, 1978). Lastly, such drugs can blunt the pleasures of life as much as the pains.

As well as drugs that influence the central nervous system, there is a vast and growing use of compounds used to regulate the peripheral parts of the autonomic nervous system. For a long time doctors have tried to sedate the gastro-intestinal system with a variety of spasmolytic agents from tincture of belladonna onwards. Of recent years we have seen a rapid increase in the use of B-blocking compounds. After the honeymoon period of enthusiasm which marks the arrival of most new drugs, we are becoming aware of their limitations and side effects. Apart from the rare complication of ocular pathology and retroperitoneal fibrosis resulting from practolol, disturbances of temperature regulation (Carruthers et al., 1974) and sexual function (Editorial, 1979) as well as a generalized lethargy have also been reported. One may also wonder about the general desirability of their widespread metabolic effects. What, for example, may be the long-term consequences of blocking the B-receptors in the what is traditionally held to be the seat of the soul, the pineal gland.

Whichever way we turn we are faced with the impossibility of achieving adequate control of the infinitely complex processes occurring within the human body by artificial external means. We must turn within to find ways of aiding the body in the magnificent feats of self-regulation achieved with the help of the autonomic nervous system.

Looking at the different methods that are available for achieving voluntary control of the involuntary nervous system, many basic similarities become apparent. This is not surprising as mankind has spent thousands of years experimenting with ways of using the same anatomical and physiological systems. These fundamental truths about "the wisdom of the body" have been discovered, rediscovered, modified to suit various patterns of living and religious beliefs, and handed down by oral tradition and in various writings. This ancient life science appears to have originated in India with various Yogic practices, spread to China, mainly in the form of Buddhism, and had been practiced in Japan as Zen meditation. Knowledge of these Eastern practices has been extremely limited in the West until this century, and only recently have the barriers of language, creed, and delusions of medical omniscience begun to break down.

Autogenic Training (AT) can probably be regarded as one of these rediscoveries of important basic principles, as it originated from research on sleep and hypnosis carried out about the turn of the century by the clinically-orientated neuropathologist, Oskar Vogt, at the Berlin Neurobiological Institute. He observed that patients who had had several sessions of hetero-hypnosis were able to put themselves in a similar state with suggestions of heaviness and warmth, and when this was repeated several times during the day, such mental exercises had remarkable restorative powers and could relieve fatigue and tension.

Johannes Schultz, who is often regarded as the father of AT, was a psychiatrist and neurologist in Berlin who began in 1905 to explore ways of extending the uses of hypnosis by reducing the passivity of the patient and his dependence on the therapist. Schultz extended Vogt's technique by instructing his patients to concentrate on sensations of heaviness and warmth in the limbs, and then adding suggestions of regularity of the heart-beat and a natural form of breathing. Because of the soothing effects of warm baths and cool compresses, Schultz then asked his subjects to think of abdominal warmth and coolness of the forehead. These six physiologically-orientated steps--heaviness and warmth in the limbs, regulation of cardiac activity and respiration, abdominal warmth and cooling of the forehead--became and remain the core of AT. The technique was progressively refined, using different verbal formula and training postures, and these are now termed the "Autogenic Standard Exercises".

The present leading exponent of AT is Dr. Wolfgang Luthe who has, appropriately enough, written the six standard books on the subject under the title of "Autogenic Therapy" (Luthe and Schultz 1969). Becoming interested in the use of AT to treat patients with bronchial asthma, Luthe developed other organ-specific exercises to treat a range of psychosomatic disorders. He later developed the idea of "intentional formula" which could be added to the basic standard exercises as a means of modifying patterns of behavior. He has also taken AT into new fields of psychotherapy with the development of abreactive techniques known as Autogenic Verbalization and Neutralization. Finally for advanced students who have learned the basic exercises and wish to extend their level of exploration of this "inner space" there is a series of meditative exercises which have many similarities with the form of Zen meditation practiced at Kyushu University, Fukuoka, Japan, where Dr. Luthe is visiting Professor of Psychophysiologic Therapy.

If meditation can be defined as "direction of attention towards an object", AT can be regarded as a Western form of meditation. In my discussion of AT, I would like to draw comparisons with one of the oldest Eastern methods of meditiation, Siddha meditation. This is an Eastern path into the interior with an ancient tradition going back thousands of years which until recently was kept a closely-guarded secret and is now being taught all over the world. (Muktananda, 1976). These simple practices give direct access to the inner conscious energy which then spontaneously powers this process of self-exploration. The changes experienced vary from a sense of well-being, understanding of life-long problems, to surges of great bliss and supreme calm. The technique has been handed down through generations of great masters to the present head of the lineage, Swami Muktananda Paramahansa. As well as relieving a wide range of emotional disorders, Siddha meditation can help in many of the clinical fields of application which I shall be describing for AT.

AT is a highly-acceptable technique because the six standard exercises can be taught progressively over a two month period with

Table 1

ANATOMY OF AUTOGENIC THERAPY

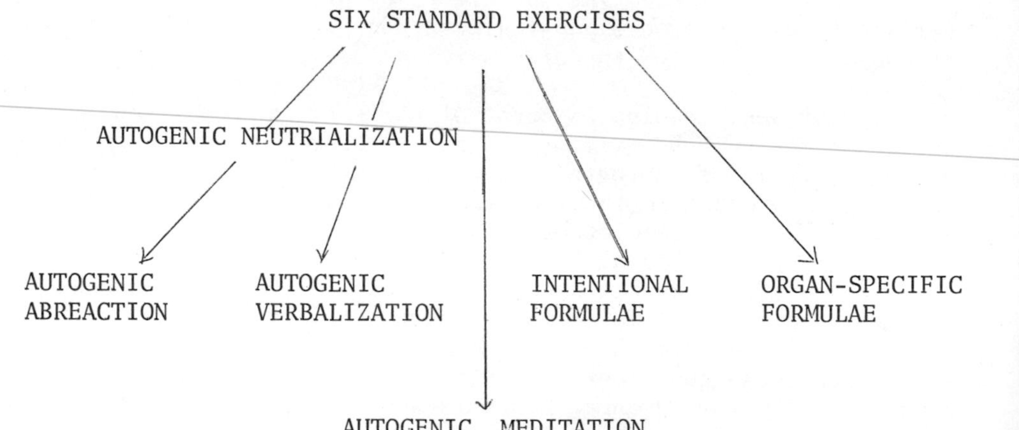

just one hour's training each week either individually or in small groups of six or eight people. Each person practices the exercises for 10 to 15 minutes two or three times every day in each of the three basic training postures, i.e. the slightly slumped standard sitting position, the armchair position, and the horizontal training position.

As one of these postures cna usually be adopted wherever the person may find themselves during the day whether in the bus, train, plane, office chair or in bed, these short practice periods can easily be built into the person's daily life and do not require their taking time off to change into practice clothing or to go anywhere special to perform the exercises. This means that AT is economic in terms of time and also of finance because unless autogenic neutralization is required for psychotherapeutic purposes, the practice requires very little of the trainer's time.

During the practice sessions the afferent stimuli are reduced as much as possible both by the stability and comfort of the posture themselves and by choosing places where noise, lighting and temperature stimuli are reduced to a minimum. With the eyes closed, the person inwardly repeats each of the verbal formula and focuses their attention on the appropriate parts of the body, the attitude being one of passive concentration. In this way, each individual progressively acquires remarkably effective voluntary control of the involuntary nervous system. During the training period there is a shift to the "autogenic state" in which the activity of the sympathetic fight and flight system is reduced. The activity of the parasympathetic rest, digest, restorative relaxation system is also increased. This achieves a readjustment of autonomic balance which, like the effects of physical training, not only acts during the exercises, but carries over to the periods between training sessions.

As well as beneficial metabolic changes, which will be discussed later in relation to the prevention and treatment of CVD, there is physiological evidence of this shift in autonomic balance with slowing of the heart-rate, reduction of blood pressure, and slowing and deepening of respiration. Also with suppression of the reticular activation system in the brain stem, cortical discharges occur which result in what are known as the "autogenic discharges". These may be either motor or sensory. The skeleto-motor discharges may cause transient twitching or jerking of the limbs, e.g. during the training sessions, while the viscera-motor discharges may be observed as increased gut sounds or salivation. The sensory discharges can include impressions of dizziness, nausea, suffocation, visual or auditory effects, or recollections of complete images or scenes, occasionally going back to very early life events.

These autogenic discharges are transient, seldom distressing, and represent a valuable unloading of brain disturbing material which has accumulated from events throughout life. This is why a detailed medical history is taken before the person starts AT to help differentiate between autogenic discharges and increased awareness of present-day pathology which results from improved communication between mind and body. This is one of many reasons why a medical presence is needed in any AT program, both to screen people entering the program and to monitor progress and training symptoms throughout. However the basic training in AT can be carried out by psychologists and psychotherapists with a wide variety of backgrounds provided there is adequate liaison with a physician who is himself trained in AT.

There are many parallels between Siddha meditation and AT. Though not requiring supervision by a doctor, meditation does require a meditation master and a properly trained teacher to guide the student. Though it is possible to meditate while lying flat or sitting comfortably in a chair a simple crossed-legged position sitting on the floor is preferable and can give the desired reduction in body awareness without allowing the person to fall asleep. Attention is focused on a specific set of sounds, the mantra, which has a similar but more generalized effect as the verbal formula in AT in progressively stilling the mind and directing attention inwards. As with the autogenic discharges, movements, or "kriyas" can occur during meditation, and there may be a wide range of sensory impressions. Both techniques however can be of great help in reducing anxiety and other neurotic symptoms as well as improving and sometimes curing a wide range of psychosomatic disorders.

The electro-encephalographic changes during AT more closely resemble those seen in meditation than the shift towards slower frequency waves and the pre-drowsy state seen either with hetero-hypnosis or autohypnosis. The changes include an increase in $\alpha$-activity, condensation of this frequency, balancing of its level in the two hemispheres, and sometimes an upward shift to the theta region.

This balancing and increased synchronisation of the two hemispheres is also claimed for techniques such as transcendental meditation. Other studies have shown that the subjective nature of the experience in AT is different from that of hypnosis, and that in AT the feelings of relaxation are more emphasized and fewer irrational feelings and sensations of disorientation were experienced (Ogawa, 1970). However these subjective impressions and the precise electrophysiologic changes seen in AT, meditation and different types of hypnosis, are likely to vary greatly from person to person and depend on their degree of experience, the conditions of the study, and the previous level of arousal or sleep deprivation. As long as each technique safely and reproducibly brings about desirable effects in the people who practice it, such technical considerations become largely of academic interest, though there is bias in the lay mind against techniques labeled "hypnotic" which are thought to involve control by outside agencies.

## APPLICATIONS OF AT

Cardiovascular disorders are often considered as having a varying underlying emotional component. Some of the factors resulting in this autonomic imbalance with a shift towards increasing sympathetic and decreasing parasympathetic activity are shown in Table 2. Significant reductions in cardiovascular risk factors such as blood pressure and blood cholesterol level have been reported with AT (Luthe and Schultz, 1969) and with other biofeedback-aided relaxation the meditation techniques (Patel and Carruthers, 1977). For the reasons already discussed, the broad spectrum of reduction in risk factors which can be obtained by such natural methods would appear to be preferable to the use of pharmacological compounds in both the primary and secondary prevention of cardiovascular disorders. AT appears to be particularly effective in the treatment of mild to moderate hypertension and brings about a profound alteration of life-style and orientation with improved adaptation to situations which would otherwise generate excessive levels of catecholamines, cortisol, and renin.

Migraine headaches also frequently respond dramatically in those cases where the triggers are more emotional than dietetic. Reduction in frequency and severity of the attacks is commonplace and people who had almost daily headaches for up to 20 years and were resistent to all known forms of therapy have been reported as totally free of the attacks by the end of the course. Such dramatic cases may be explained in the basis of decreased release of noradrenaline which may be the agent causing cerebral vasoconstriction preceding the vasodilatation which actually produces the headache (Hsu et al., 1976).

Gastro-intestinal disorders such as recurrent peptic ulceration and ulcerative colitis frequently show considerable clinical improvement on AT, and medication can often be reduced or withdrawn. The vast range of clinical disorders documented as showing improvement with AT is discussed in detail in Volume 2 of Dr. Wolfgang Luthe's reference work on Autogenic Therapy (Luthe and Schultz, 1969). There is insufficient space here to list all its applications, particularly as a deep and powerful form of psychotherapy, which is explored in Volumes 3, 5 and 6. Non-medical applications in sports, education and industry are also extensive. To summarize however, I should like to suggest that non-drug techniques such as AT and Siddha meditation will come to be appreciated as having a valuable part to play in the prevention and treatment of disease, and that in many clinical situations "meditation not medication" should be our motto.

Table 2. Autonomic Factors in Cardiovascular Disease

| | SYMPATHETIC DOMINANCE | PARASYMPATHETIC DOMINANCE |
|---|---|---|
| PROMOTING FACTORS | STRESS | PHYSICAL TRAINING |
| | (Emotional, Physical, Thermal) | MENTAL TRAINING |
| | SURGERY | (Autogenic Training and Yoga) |
| | SMOKING | SLEEP |
| METABOLIC EFFECTS | CATABOLIC | ANABOLIC |
| TESTOSTERONE AND INSULIN | DECREASED | INCREASED |
| FIBRINOLYTIC ACTIVITY | DECREASED | INCREASED |
| CATECHOLAMINES AND CORTICOSTEROIDS | INCREASED | DECREASED |
| LIPIDS, GLUCOSE + URIC ACID | INCREASED | DECREASED |
| HEART RATE + BLOOD PRESSURE | INCREASED | DECREASED |
| SIGNS AND SYMPTOMS OF TISSUE HYPOXIA | INCREASED | DECREASED |
| (e.g. angina, limb pain, ST-T depression) | | |

REFERENCES

Carruthers, M. E., Taggart, P., Salpekar, P. D., and Gatt, J. A., 1974, Some metabolic effects of beta-blockade on temperature regulation and in the presence of trauma, in "Beta-blockers--Present Status and Future Prospects," W. Schweizer, ed., Hans Huber, Berne.

Clayton, A. B., 1976, The effects of psychotropic drugs upon driving-related skills, Human Factors, 18:241.

Editorial, 1979, Drugs and male sexual function, Brit. Med. Jnl., 2:883.

Gordon, B., 1979, "I'm Dancing as Fast as I Can," Harper and Row, New York.

Hawkins, F. H., 1978, "Sleep and Body Rhythm Disturbance in Long-Range Aviation," Monograph, Churchill Fellowship Study, Winston Churchill Memorial Trust, London.

Horrobin, D. F., Ghayur, T., and Karmali, R. A., 1979, Mind and cancer, letter to Lancet, 1:978.

Hsu, L. K. G., Crisp, A. H., Kalucy, R. S., Koval, J., Chen, C. N., Carruthers, M. E., Zilkha, K. J., 1976, Early morning migraine, Lancet, 1:447.

Illich, I., 1975, "Medical Nemesis," Calder and Boyars Ltd., London.

Kochansky, G. E., Salzman, C., Shader, R. I., Harmatz, J. S., and Ogoltree, A. M., 1977, Effects of chlordiazepoxide and oxazepam administration on verbal hostility, Arch. of Gen. Psychia., 34:1457.

Luthe, W., and Schultz, J. H., 1969, "Autogenic Therapy," Grune and Stratton, New York.

Muktananda, P., 1976, "Play of Consciousness," Harper and Row, New York.

Ogawa, K., 1970, Differences between hypnosis and autogenic training: A factor-analytical study, Jap. Jnl. of Hyp., 15:14.

Patel, C., and Carruthers, M. E., 1977, Coronary risk factor reduction through biofeedback-aided relaxation and meditation, Jnl. of the Roy. Col. of Gen. Pract., 27:401.

Salzman, C., Kochansky, G. E., Shader, R. I., Porrino, L. J., Harmatz, J. S., and Swett, C. P., 1974, Chlordiazepoxide induced hostility in a small group setting, Arch. of Gen. Psychia., 31:401.

Skegg, D. C., Richards, S. M., and Doll, R., 1979, Minor tranquilizers and road accidents, Brit. Med. Jnl., 1:917.

# EXPERIMENTS IN TENSION CONTROL

# TENSION CONTROL: DIFFERENCES BETWEEN SUBJECTS INSTRUCTED IN PROGRESSIVE RELAXATION OR PLACEBO CONTROL SESSIONS

Marcella Woods, Ph.D.

Director, Tension Control Center
Seattle, Washington

Within the past fifteen years a number of studies has focused on the psychophysiological role of awareness in the apprehension and control of muscle tension, as well as, whether or not training in a specific modality enhances awareness. Investigations in progressive relaxation, biofeedback training, and autogenic training, have led to contradictory findings.[1-12] The contradictions appear to occur at several levels. At the psychophysiological level the question arises, "Does conscious awareness play a significant role in the voluntary control of muscle tension?" At the measurement level the problem becomes, by what technique does one measure awareness?

The defining and observing of awareness pose problems in measurement as was pointed out by Sime.[10] In his study he sought to eliminate the confounding effect of feedback, which was present in the Kinsman, et al., study,[8] by excluding feedback from the testing procedures. In so doing Sime's data analyses supported the assumption that with training, i.e., biofeedback or progressive relaxation, subjects are able to accurately judge in some instances muscle tension in gross qualitative terms of "more" or "less than." The contention, therefore, is that in the absence of feedback, subjects' awareness was dependent upon attention to a somatic cue and that the primary cue was muscle tension, per se.

This does not necessarily follow. That awareness was demonstrated is not questioned. It is the nature or specificity of awareness that is questionable. To conclude that muscle tension per se comprised the cue-content is not justified since other somatic cues were available. Research designs with respect to the aforementioned studies have not controlled for such somatic cues as cutaneous and thermal, or for the subjective sensation of fatigue. Admittedly, control of these cues poses problems.

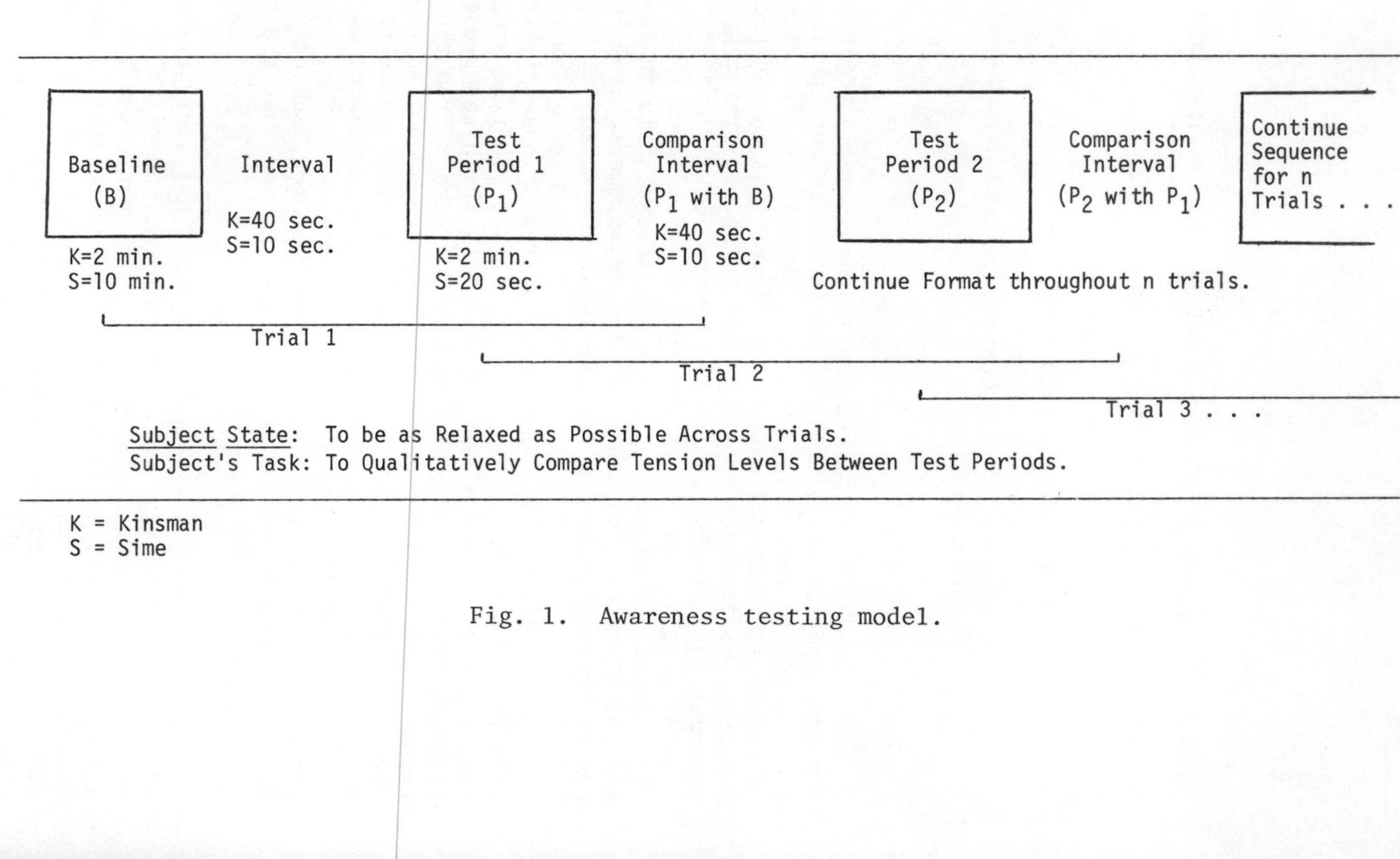


Fig. 1. Awareness testing model.

Of further concern is the confounding of data that can occur as a result of subjects' skill in recall. The function of recall of contraction effort necessary for activation of a selected motor unit(s) under distracting influences was alluded to by Wagman and his colleagues.[13] Skill in recall appears to be ignored by investigators but might be central to studies that purport to investigate the awareness factor relative to the control of skeletal muscle tension.

To illustrate the likelihood of a recall skill variable, consider the Kinsman[8] model depicted below. It is apparent that approximately five minutes separated each comparison interval. In Sime's study, the elapsed time beginning test period 1 through the comparison interval following test period 2 was reduced to approximately one minute. It is conceivable that recall skill, if it is a critcal variable, might have been less for one minute than for five minutes.

Since the majority of these awareness studies have required a subjective/cognitive evaluation of performance, the subjects have been put into a paradoxical situation. On the one hand they are directed to, "relax as much as possible," and on the other hand, informed that their task is to compare/evaluate their own status at the end of a defined period. In order to compare/evaluate one must remain alert. But to remain so requires that one selectively attend to a given type of information for a period of time, that one be able to discriminate alteration of that information, that one be able to integrate/synthesize that selected information flow into a sense or impression of what is occurring or did occur.

To accomplish awareness necessitates some level of concentration. Concentration requires effort, and underlying effort is tension. It appears that subjects are placed in an impossible to perform situation. Does this not occur to them at some point during the testing? If so, does this provoke anxiety or feelings of discomfort? Should the answer to these questions be in the affirmative, then it is conceivable that subjects are reporting comparisons in their discomfort states rather than their awareness of muscle tension at a specific site (e.g., frontalis). This presents a type of locus-focus hocus-pocus set of circumstances. The point of the foregoing discussion is that until studies are designed to control for the utilization of other available somatic cues, to investigate the influence of recall skill with such fleeting, subtle and random events as muscle-action potentials, and then to control for inter-subject differences the role and specificity of awareness only can remain unresolved.

Rather than wrestle with the problems besetting awareness testing, it seemed that a more productive approach would be to investigate at the somatic rather than cognitive level the discrimination of signaling. For all the other things that it might be, tension control is fundamentally motor precision.

The search for mechanisms involved in accomplishing motor precision has led to numerous studies utilizing the feedback model. However, in fitting this cybernetic machine model to a living biological system it appears investigators have lost sight of the fact that feedback is a negative or error-correcting program. It is an argument of this paper that while feedback is necessary to the correction of motor acts gone astray and provides reinforcement for well executed motor acts, it is of equal import to investigate input. The work of Festinger and Canon[15] demonstrated that over and above the afferent feedback we usually get as a result of an efferent, we can be aware of our efference. Through their visual-spatial localization experiments they were able to show that we do make use of "outflow information" from the motor and pre-motor cortex. It would seem, therefore, that tension control, in effecting the relaxation of skeletal muscle, might be accomplished by inhibition of the montoneurons that excite it. This would have to occur since in relaxed musculature of sub-microvoltage levels there appears to be virtual elimination of proprioceptive feedback. In the case of directing subjects to relax the frontalis musculature, if successful, the experience of tension should be non-existent since technically there would be no recognizable proprioceptive signals. If the frontalis is consciously relaxed, i.e., electrical silence $\leq$ 1.0, uV, then the only information that might be available would be that of the inhibitory efferents from the cortex blocking the efferents that usually innervate the musculature. Therefore efferent control, that is input, rather than afferent feedback might be more critical in both the creation of appropriate tension necessary for motor precision in human efforts as well as in relaxation of musculature. The finding by Basmajian that control over the discharge of a motor unit during proximal and distal joint movements "requires a great mental concentration on the motor activity" appears to offer support to the critical nature of input control.[14]

Keeping in mind that tension control as a function of appropriate input is a subtle but complex neuromuscular skill, an assessment model that engages the subject in performing as closely as possible to the manner in which we perform daily was developed in 1976. The focus therefore was to demonstrate control by doing, rather than by reporting one's impressions of the qualities of a past event.

To test control in this manner, the assessment model was designed with the following assumptions:

1. That awareness of somatic activity would be occurring during the active or tensing phase; thus, to use Merton's term, a "sense of effort"[17] would be generated.

2. During the relaxation phase of tension control one would assume that if relaxation occurred, there would be an absense of afferent signaling; therefore, awareness would be non-

existent unless efferents ceased to be inhibited, whereupon, a "sense of effort" would occur.

3. During the active or tensing period of the testing model, the subject would have to attend to the tension she would be generating, and manage control on the basis of efferent outflow (input) in order to achieve the intended contraction of muscle fibers. On the basis of this assumption a subject skilled in consciously controlling tension generation should be able to create tension in a specific muscle (e.g., frontalis) at a level approximating minimal tension (i.e., 10 uV) in a consistent manner over a number of trials.* Since there was no prior practice in creating minimum tension levels and all performance occurred in the absence of external feedback, the assumptions prevail that the subjects attend to somatic cues and performance is not a function of recall (memory).

4. During the pre-contraction stages of the tension period, skilled subjects would be able to minimize their action-potential levels in a situation that ordinarily would elicit anticipatory tension (AT).

5. During post-contraction ($P\text{-}C_{1,2}$) stages of the tensing period and during the two relaxtion periods subjects skilled in tension control would be able to achieve electrical silence ($\leq$ 1.0 uV).

These foregoing assumptions were tested and these results were reported at the 1977 AAATC meeting in Chicago, Illinois, USA, at which time the Woods Tension Control Assessment protocol was introduced.* Presented were data supporting the sensitivity of the protocol for the assessment of tension control. The research presented in this report represents a continuation of investigations utilizing the protocol in which the following null hypothesis was tested:

> There is no difference in tension control skill as measured by the Woods protocol between a Placebo Control (PC) group and subjects trained for 8-weeks (16 instructional sessions) in Progressive Relaxation (PR).

---

*Rationale presented in report given at the American Association for the Advancement of Tension Control (AAATC) meeting in Chicago, Illinois, 1977.

*Complete description and standardized instructions are available and may be requested from the author.

To reject the above hypothesis it was determined a priori that the following sub-hypotheses would have to be rejected at $p \leq .05$.

1. There is no difference in skill between PR trained and PC groups to reproduce self-initiated minimum tension.

2. There is no difference in skill between PR trained and PC groups in relaxing a selected skeletal muscle.

3. There is no difference in skill between PR trained and PC groups in minimizing anticipatory tension.

## METHODS

### Subjects

Sixty females having a mean age of 38.4 years were selected from a pool of women who answered an advertisement for free evaluation of natural skill in tension control and an opportunity to improve their skill. Those selected qualified for inclusion by meeting the following criteria:

1. Not under treatment for functional tension disorders.

2. Not under treatment for pathological disease.

3. Not on mind altering drugs or medication, other than an occasional aspirin.

4. No previous experience with formal instruction in progressive relaxation or other tension control techniques.

Occupational classifications represented were those of homemaker, professional, technical, and secretarial.

### Prodedures

All selected subjects were individually orientated to the assessment program and evaluated in accordance with the Woods protocol. Frontalis EMG using standard placement was monitored with silver-silver chloride surface electrodes and the Jacobson Integrating Neuro-voltmeter. Skin to electrode resistance was kept to 2K Ohms or below. Data were collected while subjects were in a semi-reclining position, were in the post-absorptive state, and had ingested no alcohol or caffeine products within two hours of data collection. Subjects who were smokers were instructed to refrain from smoking for two hours prior to testing. All subjects affirmed they had followed instructions.

Subjects were pre-tested only once, since an unpublished study conducted by Woods had indicated no significant difference in performance after 7 days or 10 weeks re-test intervals in the absence of formal instruction. After pre-test data were processed, each subject received a copy of her tension-control profile indicating her strengths and weaknesses.

Both groups engaged in an eight weeks program consisting of two 60 minute instructional sessions per week and instructions for daily practice (7 days/week). Subjects in both groups submitted daily practice logs. The only experimenter-manipulated variable between the two groups' experiences was that which occurred during the two 60 minute instructional sessions per week.

PR group: Instruction in the recognition, production, and release of muscular tension in the specific muscle or muscle group presentation sequence designed by Jacobson, outlined in the 1964 manual entitled, Self-Operations Control.

PC group: The control subjects were instructed to direct their attention to a particular muscle or group and determine whether or not there was any sensation of effort/tension present; if detected, to release. If a sensation of effort was not detected, they were to remain released. Attention was to be directed at a frequency which seemed to the subject to be 20 seconds beyond the previous period of attending. Muscle control sites were presented in the same sequence as for the PR group.

At the end of each instructional session both groups were reminded to refrain from engaging in new activities or habits for the remainder of the eight week period. To control for subjects attempting to meet the experimenter's expectations or deceiving the experimenter, subjects were encouraged to discuss any change in their lifestyle from the status quo with the experimenter to ascertain whether the event or its continuance would affect one's progress in tension control skill development.

Within one to two weeks following the cessation of the eight-week instructional program, subjects from both groups were retested at the same time of day as initial testing. Thus, time of day was controlled. To control for possible decay in skill, subjects from each group were randomly assigned to either week 1 or week 2 for the post instruction testing.

## RESULTS

Skill in tension control was assessed before and after eight weeks of progressive relaxation instruction or placebo control, using the Woods Tension Control Assessment protocol. Pre-experiment data supported the null regarding differences between groups. The techniques of constant error (CE) and variable error (VE) were applied to determine each subject's control profile, and both groups' mean performances with respect to each element of the protocol are illustrated in Figures 2 and 3.

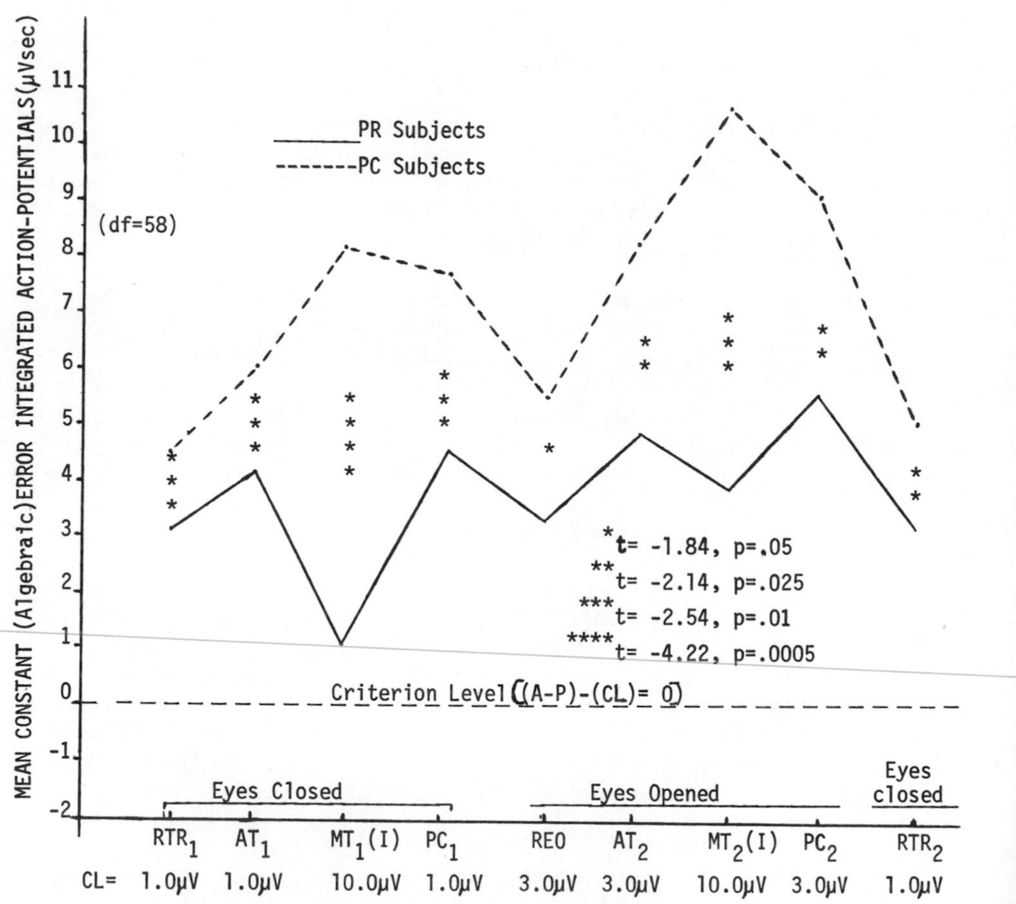


Fig. 2. Post-instruction criterion performance between subjects instructed in progressive relaxation and subjects assigned to placebo instruction.

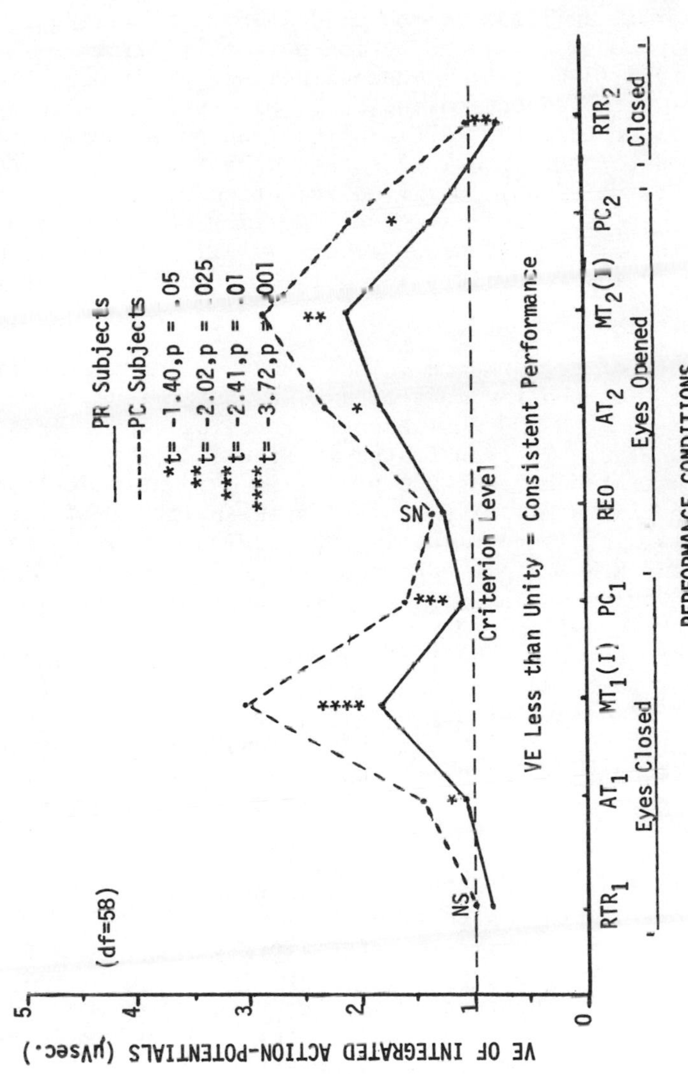


Fig. 3. Post-instruction performance consistency between subjects instructed in progressive relaxation and subjects assigned to placebo instruction.

Data displayed in Figure 2 represent both differences and similarities of action-potentials (A-P) recorded relative to criterion levels (CL) following the 8 weeks of PR or PC sessions. Thus one aspect of tension control skill is hypothesized as being the ability to perform at criterion microvoltage levels that are physiologically premised. Studies, heretofore, have utilized a percentage of a practiced, arbitrarily selected, force production. Achieving criterion performance may be expressed as action-potentials minus criterion level equals zero (A-P-CL=0). Whereas neither group achieved criterion level A-Ps with respect to the skill elements assessed by the protocol, it is clear that the PR group's action-potentials were more closely related to criterion-levels than were those of the PC group. One-tailed t-tests (df=58) justified rejection of the null for each skill element, thereby, indicating the ability of the PR group to either generate or reduce tension levels in all performance measures at significantly lower levels than could be accomplished by the PC group.

Consistency of performance in each skill element constitutes the second component of tension control and was determined through variable error (VE). $VE \leq 1.0$ was accepted as being consistent performance. Akin to Figure 2, illustrated in Figure 3 is the degree of consistency demonstrated by each group. It is evident that both groups may be described as similarly consistent in ability to maintain action-potential levels (A-P) during the residual tension reduction states ($RTR_1$ and $RTR_2$). Although demonstrated is a significant difference between the means at $RTR_2$ it perhaps becomes frivolous to quibble over the question, "How consistent is consistent?" Otherwise, as one examines Figure 3, the skill elements, $RTR_1$, resting with eyes open (REO), and post-contraction ($P-C_2$) are the elements for which the hypothesis of no difference between the groups was accepted. Thus, the significant t-tests strongly suggest that while not achieving criterion consistency in seven of the nine elements, the PR group did demonstrate a greater degree of stability during performance than did the PC subjects.

On the basis of these data, those instructed in progressive relaxation performed with a significantly lower constant error (CE) and a significantly greater degree of stability (VE) than did the placebo control subjects. Further, this tendency generalized across six of the nine elements of the protocol to the extent that one may conclude evidence exists for stating that with eight weeks of systematic instruction in progressive relaxation, subjects will develop tension control skill levels that significantly exceed those of a placebo-instruction group.

## DISCUSSION

The uniqueness of this study resides in its conceptual and measurement approaches that are departures from studies previously reported. At the conceptual level, skill in tension control is considered as control of input (i.e., efferent outflow from the motor and pre-motor cortex that is subjectively experienced as effort) rather than informational feedback. Control of input does not preclude the necessity for feedback but conceptually and experientially shifts the focus of control from that which has occurred to that which is about to occur or is occurring. As performance, this shift engages the subject in initiating for motor precision rather than correcting that which was poorly initiated. Thus it is presumed that greater efficiency in effort-to-task matching will be the result of improved input control.

As a measurement strategy, it was reasoned that engaging the subject in initiating all elements of control fundamental to skilled tension control would be a more productive approach to assessing skill. That by doing, one demonstrates the skill one has at a given point in time, under a given set of circumstances, and that measurement of one's doing, rather than one's reporting on what one has done, evaluates at the experience level rather than at the cognitive/subjective (self-report) level. Measuring at the experience level removes the frequently-observed lack of congruence between what one has done and what one believes to have done. It is hypothesized that in the absence of external feedback the subject is forced to attend to somatic cues that bring about the sensation or feeling that one is in control. Specifically this is believed to occur during those periods within the protocol that one is to reproduce a qualitative amount (i.e., minimum) of tension* and then to voluntarily release to pre-tension levels. During those periods in which the subject is to remain relaxed (i.e., residual neuromuscular action-potentials $\leq$ 1.0 uV), when ordinarily one would be generating anticipatory tension, it is further hypothesized that the ability to relax by letting-go or discontinuing efferent input contributes to the sense/feeling of control.

Because of the control of extraneous variables identified earlier in this study, the use of a placebo control situation that approximated instructional sessions, and the data generated through the use of an assessment protocol that treats tension control as a measurable neuromuscular skill rather than a subjective awareness or recall (memory) exercise, the following new hypotheses for a theory of tension control as motor precision are offered.

1. Tension control is a measurable neuromuscular skill that is

*Unknown to the subject is the criterion level of 10 uV.

conditioned by the development of more precise motor input.

2. Tension control is a function of the ability to sense different effort (tension) levels, to reproduce these levels when that is the task/objective, and to release tension to lower levels all in a consistent manner. To do so suggests that one has developed less labile tension habits.

3. Development of skilled tension control performance cannot be achieved through placebo instruction sessions.

4. Long term instruction in progressive relaxation combined with assessing tension control that is learned as a neuromuscular skill, offer a more productive approach to determining the efficacy of progressive relaxation as prevention of tension disorders or as treatment. Unless it can be demonstrated that one has learned or developed skill in tension control, any discussion addressing efficacy of treatment or as prevention of tension/stress-related disorders may be premature with any given subject, patient, or client.

The design of this study eliminated such contaminating variables as recall skill and subjective/cognitive evaluations that might relate to discomfort states rather than sensitivity to tension or effort signals.

Unresolved by this study was the question of cue-content. It is concluded that somatic cues were the choice attentional efforts. However, it cannot be stated that muscle tension per se constituted the performance information set. Throughout this study the subject's ability to monitor input (efferent outflow), rather than feedback, has been suggested as the cue-content necessary for achieving and demonstrating the kind of motor precision that is required for tension control.

Until studies are undertaken to tease out the cue-content, one cannot be certain how one achieves conscious tension control. In the meantime the hypothesis is advanced that to develop skill in tension control through progressive relaxation, it is necessary during the learning stage to engage in experiences that direct attention to input. In so doing, the learner increases sensitivity to the efforts that are being produced relative to the task for which the tension/efforts are being generated with respect to the desired outcome. Therefore, as control of input increases, one develops more tension control and exhibits the fine tuning that can be recognized as motor precision.

REFERENCES


1. E. Jacobson, "Teaching and Learning," National Foundation for Progressive Relaxation, Chicago (1973).
2. B. A. Pearse, E. D. Walter, J. D. Sergent and M. Meers, Exploratory observations of the use of an intensive autogenic biofeedback training procedure in a follow-up study of out-of-town patients having migraine and/or tension headache, Unpublished paper given at the Biofeedback Research meeting, (February, 1975).
3. P. Grimm, "Relaxation, Meditation and Insight," cited by W. E. Sime in "Proceedings of the Second Annual Meeting of the American Association for the Advancement of Tension Control," F. J. McGuigan, ed., University Publications, Blacksburg, Va. (1975).
4. S. Rachman, The role of muscular relaxation in densitization therapy, Behav. Res. and Ther., 6:159 (1968).
5. A. Gessel, Biofeedback-enhanced training in therapeutic muscular relaxation: A clinician's view, in "Proceedings of the First Annual Meeting of the American Association for the Advancement of Tension Control," F. J. McGuigan, ed., University Publications, Blacksburg, Va. (1974).
6. I. Matus, Internal awareness, muscle sense and muscle relaxation in bioelectric information feedback training, cited by W. E. Sime in "Proceedings of the Second Annual Meeting of the American Association for the Advancement of Tension Control," F. J. McGuigan, ed., University Publications, Blacksburg, Va. (1975).
7. W. E. Sime, Psychophysiology of muscle tension relaxation: A comparative study of EMG biofeedback and autosensory feedback relaxation training, (personal communication).
8. R. A. Kinsman, K. O'Banion, S. Robinson, and H. Staudenmayer, Continuous biofeedback and discrete post-trial verbal feedback in frontalis muscle relaxation training, Psychophys., 12:30 (1975).
9. D. S. Chaney and L. Andreasen, Relaxation and neuromuscular tension control and changes in motor performance under induced tension, Percept. and Mot. Skills, 36:185, (1973).
10. W. E. Sime, Role of awareness in muscle tension relaxation, in "Proceedings of the Second Annual Meeting of the American Association for the Advancement of Tension Control, F. J. McGuigan, ed., University Publications, Blacksburg, Va. (1975).
11. R. Rummel, Electromyographic analysis of patterns used to reproduce muscular tension, Res. Quart. 3:64 (1974).
12. D. E. Shedivy and K. M. Kleinman, Lack of correlation between frontalis EMG and either neck EMG or verbal ratings of tension, Psychophys., 14:182, (1977).

13. I. H. Wagman, D. S. Pierce and R. E. Burger, Proprioceptive influence in volitional control of individual motor units, Nature, 207:957, (1965).
14. J. B. Basmajian, Microcosmic learning single nerve-cell training, in "Proceedings of the Committee on Institutional Cooperation Symposium on Psychology of Motor Learning," L. E. Smith, ed., Athletics Institute, Chicago, (1969).
15. L. Festinger and L. K. Canon, Information about spatial location based on knowledge about efference, Psych. Rev., 72:373 (1965).
16. T. C. Ruch, H. D. Patton, J. W. Woodbury and A. L. Towe, "Neurophysiology," Saunders and Co., Philadelphia (1961).
17. P. A. Merton, How we control the contraction of our muscles, Sci., 5:30 (1972).

# THE MODIFICATION OF THE HORMONAL AND METABOLIC EFFECTS OF MENTAL STRESS BY PHYSICAL EXERCISE

Richard A. Graveling, Ph.D.

Head of Basic Studies, Human Sciences
Ergonomics Branch
Institute of Occupational Medicine
Staffordshire, England

The work described in this paper was carried out when the author was employed at the University of Salford, Human Performance Laboratory, under a research fellowship from the Leverhulme Trust, whose help is gratefully acknowledged.

The concept of stress is one which is currently much used, or possibly misused. Its definition has frequently been the subject of discussion in the scientific literature, perhaps highlighted in the papers by Mason and Selye in the Journal of Human Stress in 1975, and those which subsequently appeared in the book edited by Serban in 1976. However, such discussions tend to be rather time-consuming and must be omitted from this paper. I have adopted a working definition of stress as the total environmental load (internal and external) and the stress response as all responses, both specific and non-specific, made to that load.

Physical activity is frequently regarded as being 'good for you' not only in terms of cardio-respiratory fitness but also for general health and well-being. Kenneth Cooper referred to exercise as having a tension-releasing function in that, if carried out in the late afternoon or early evening, it left one relaxed for the duration of the evening. However, he subsequently introduced an element of contradiction, stating that it was inadvisable to go to bed immediately after strenuous exercise as the body needed a chance to "unwind" for at least an hour prior to sleep.

Scientific studies of this proposed beneficial effect of exercise are scarce. De Vries reported a study where exercise produced a greater degree of muscular relaxation than a single dose of a

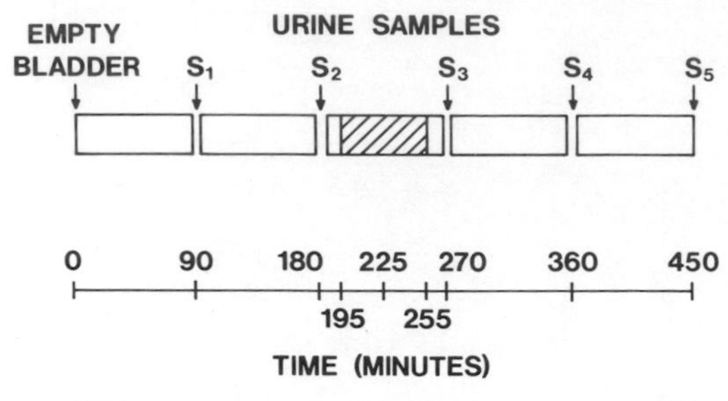


Fig. 1. Experimental design used in experiment

tranquilizer, as measured by electromyography, but little other work has been found.

Some apparently contradictory evidence can, however, be drawn from the literature. A number of authors, including Taggart and colleagues, and Frankenhaeuser, have referred to the apparent relationship between repeated or prolonged elevations in plasma levels of the catecholamines--adrenaline and noradrenaline--and potentially pathological states. Similarly, mental stress is frequently blamed as a cause of such elevated levels and thus, indirectly, impairing health. However, exercise has <u>also</u> been shown to increase plasma catecholamine concentrations, apparently contradicting claims for beneficial effects.

The study described briefly here was set up to carry out a preliminary investigation of whether exercise can reduce the potentially harmful effects of mental stress.

The mental work task used was a multichoice reaction time task, operating in two sensory modes, which had previously been shown to produce significant changes in excretion patterns of some hormonal products (Thomason et al., 1977).

Clearly, any beneficial effect of exercise on well-being or tension control may result from psychological factors associated with sports participation rather than the mechanical aspects of exercise. However, as the experimental control of the intensity of exercise was considered to be an important factor in evaluating hormonal responses, 'laboratory type' exercise on a cycle ergometer was chosen. The workload was set for each subject to represent 60-70 percent of his maximum aerobic capacity.

Eight healthy male subjects took part in the experiment. Figure 1 shows the experimental design used. Subjects collected all urine passed during the day according to this schedule.

**TREATMENTS**

A – REST + EXERCISE

B – MENTALWORK + REST

C – REST + REST (CONTROL)

D – MENTALWORK + EXERCISE

Fig. 2. Experimental sessions were each made up of two 30-minute blocks.

They were all members of staff at the University of Salford and carried out their normal duties during most of the day with the exception of the central period when they attended the laboratory on site (a maximum of five minutes walk from their workplace).

Each experimental session was made up of two-30 minute blocks as shown in Figure 2.

Each subject carried out each experimental treatment once according to two 4 by 4 latin squares.

Urine samples were analyzed using a multi-hormonal chromatographic analysis. They were separately analyzed for 17 oxogenic steroids. The development and procedures for analysis have been described elsewhere (Bark et al., 1977).

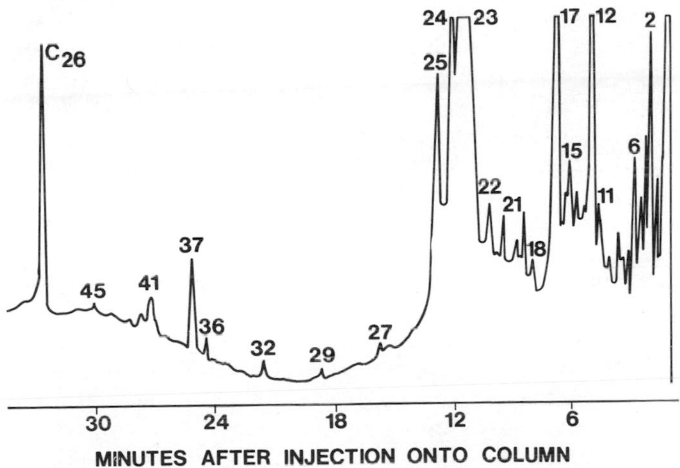


Fig. 3. Diagram of a urinary metabolic profile from the gas chromatograph.

## RESULTS AND DISCUSSION

Figure 3 shows a typical chromatographic trace. Each peak represents a separate component and the height of the peak provides a measure of concentration.

Urinary excretion rates calculated from such traces were analyzed statistically using the Wilcoxon Rank Test for paired observations using probability levels of .05 and .01.

In the present study, nine of the compounds, not all of which have been identified, demonstrated statistically significant changes due to treatments. In addition, the separate analysis of 17-oxogenic steroids showed a significant effect.

Limits of time do not permit me to present these results in detail but the trends described are all supported by the statistical analysis.

The exercise task alone increased the excretion rate of most of the 10 compounds showing significant effects including vanillic acid and vanilmandelic acid (metabolites of adrenaline and noradrenaline) and homovanillic acid from dopamine. In the case of the 3 compounds where this significant increase did not occur, the exercise task apparently prevented the significant decrease which occurred on the control day. This can be interpreted as an increase in excretion compared to basal levels. For example, on the control day there was a significant fall in the 17-oxogenic steroid excretion rate across the afternoon but no such fall occurred on the exercise treatment day.

The pattern of results in response to the mental work task was much less clear cut. Two compounds showed a significant increase in excretion rate following the mental work task, and several others showed an increase relative to basal levels, that is not demonstrating the significant decrease shown on the control day, (for example, hippuric acid). Other compounds, including those from the catecholamines, did not show any changes different to those on the control day. This lack of uniformity of response, unlike that produced by the physical exercise, was probably a function of the complexity of mental stress and is seen as support for a multi-hormonal analytical approach such as that adopted here, rather than examining isolated hormonal systems.

The treatment involving physical exercise following mental work demonstrated a number of differing effects. One which was very clear was the interaction between the effects of the two differing forms of stress. No compound showed any indication of an accumulative effect.

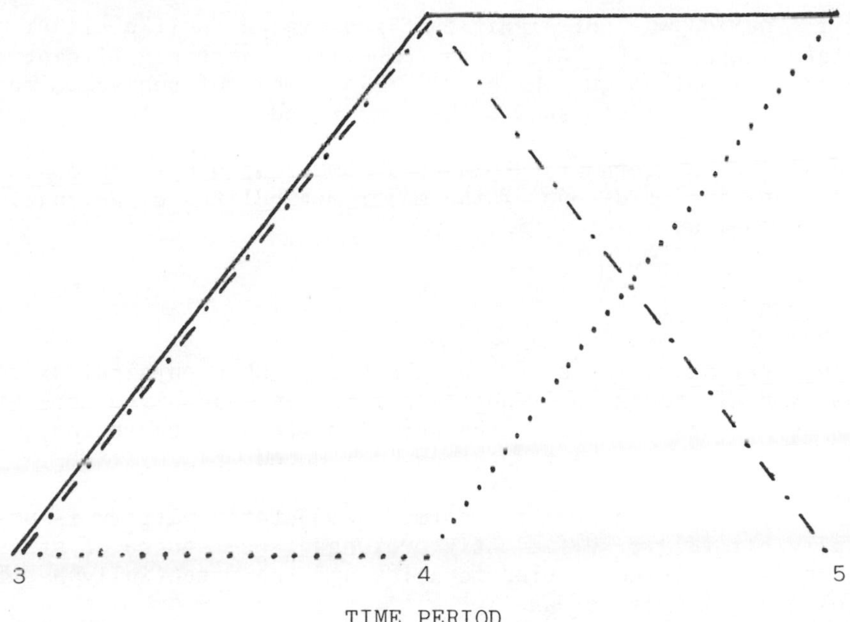


Fig. 4. Pattern of statistically significant changes.

——— A $3 < 4$; $3 < 5$; $p = .01$

· · · · · B $3 < 5$; $p = .01$

— · — D $3 < 4$; $p = .01$

The responses could be divided into three main groups. In the first, no apparent interaction occurred. This was demonstrated as an effect due to physical exercise which was not modified by the inclusion of mental work. The second was a generalized stress response with all three threatments showing a common pattern which differed from that of the control day. The third was the interaction such that the effects of one or both of the sources of stress was reduced by the combination of the two.

For example, the excretion rate for the compound represented in Figure 4 was significantly elevated by exercise alone, and remained elevated during the final period in comparison to time period 3.

With mental work alone, the increase in excretion rate did not attain statistical significance over time period 3 until the fifth period.

However, when the two treatments were combined, although the initial response followed that of exercise, the excretion rate during the fifth period was not significantly elevated, unlike either treatment taken separately. All these comparisons were significant at a probability level of .01 which, for this number of subjects, means that all eight subjects showed the same trend.

A similar pattern was shown by a number of other compounds including vanillic acid, one of the major metabolites of adrenaline and noradrenaline.

## CONCLUSIONS

In conclusion, the study has shown that when physical exercise follows mental stress the tendency for the individual sources of stress to produce changes in the normal pattern of excretion, as shown by the control treatment, can be reduced.

As any deviation from the normal homeostatic pattern is potentially harmful if sufficiently prolonged, one source of stress can, therefore, be considered to alleviate the potentially harmful physiological effects of another.

This finding only directly relates to the specific situation under which the study was carried out. Further work is necessary to investigate whether this conclusion can be considered to have a wider applicability. Nevertheless, the clear cut existence of interactive effects is very interesting and clearly warrants further investigation.

The results also demonstrate the need to examine the human responses to stress as a functional entity rather than studying individual hormonal systems in isolation.

## REFERENCES

Bark, L. S., Graveling, R. A., and Thomason, H., 1977, Some applications of gas-liquid chromatography in the investigation of the relationship between physiological stress and physical activity, Proceed. of the Analyt. Div. of the Chem. Soc., 14:248.

Mason, J. W., 1975, A historical view of the stress field, Jnl. of Hum. Stress, 1:6.

Selye, H., 1975, Confusion and controversy in the stress field, Jnl. of Hum. Stress, 1:37.

Serban, G., (ed.), 1975, "Psychopathology of Human Adaptation," Plenum, New York.

Thomason, H., Graveling, R. A., Bark, L. S., and Hamley, E. J., 1977, The analysis of multi-hormonal responses of the human to changes in environment, Unpublished presentation, 27th International Congress of Physiological Sciences, Paris.

# THE LIFE OF EDMUND JACOBSON

# EDMUND JACOBSON -- PIONEER AND "FATHER" OF TENSION CONTROL AND PROGRESSIVE RELAXATION

Endre Szirmai, M.D., Ph.D.

Chairman, Department of Nuclear Hematology
Institute of Nuclear Energy
Stuttgart, West Germany

As Seneca, the Roman writer once said, "In life as in a drama it is not important how long, but how well it was acted".

Regarding Edmund Jacobson, our great president, we can say that he has been acting very well and very long. He made his great progress using his new ideas and realizing them, partly in collaboration with his colleagues. During his long lifetime Edmund Jacobson inspired not only one but several new generations by his experimental and practical work. Our great friend may well be called the "father" of tension control and progressive relaxation.

His effect was all the greater by team-work in different frontier fields of science. The results of his researches were presented at several national and international conferences and congresses and were published in journals as well as in proceedings and textbooks.

An outstanding event for Edmund and for us was in the fall 1974 when on October 12 and 13 the American Association for the Advancement of Tension Control was founded in Bismarck Hotel, Chicago, Illinois. Professor F. J. McGuigan also plays an important role in this AAATC. At this conference specialists from different countries reported on their experiences in the field mentioned which Edmund Jacobson had already worked out and described in the present form in 1924.

There were many publications on Edmund and his great achievements in many journals. Let me mention just two as examples: "Pain in the Neck is all in Your Head" wrote George Alexander in the Los Angeles Times, and "Mr. Relaxation is Honored" was reported in another paper.

All of us know the books Edmund wrote, we know about his success in treating nervous tension and in clarifying problems in this connection. It would take me a long time, I think, not only half an hour or so, but some days, to specify the steps of Edmund's work, his writings, his career. I have written a chapter about him and though it is rather long it is merely a short summary compared to the bulk of what he achieved.

I do agree with Enrico Fermi whose colleague Eugene P. Wigner is, by the way, a good friend of mine.

"The greatest enemy of science is not ignorance but half-knowledge". Edmund Jacobson removed vague knowledge in a field so far unexplored; he gave us valuable new knowledge.

But here I am not going to talk about science itself but about a man deeply engaged in science and thus having become a part of the history of science.

Born 91 years ago, Edmund Jacobson has not only been witness of most important events but has, directly and indirectly, influenced them, devoting himself to problems of national affairs.

Time being short I must omit most of the interesting connections Edmund had with a large number of well-known men and women, among them the Nobel Laureate Charles B. Huggins, Admiral Nimitz, the Presidents Roosevelt and Truman, Aldous Huxley, Alfred Adler and many more.

Here I am quoting passages from Edmund's letters which will give you a lively impression of what he did and who he is:

"I hope that the following account will provide the information kindly requested in your letter... In 1864, at the age of 12, my father, Morris Jacobson, came to America from Strasbourg, which was then in France, as it is now. His forefathers, I believe, had emigrated from Denmark, whence the name..."

"In 1883 he left Michigan to come to Chicago where he met my mother, Frances Blum, aged 16, when they became engaged. Four years later they were married. My father's business in Chicago developed into real estate buying and selling... My mother's father had emigrated from Berlin in 1848 to Des Moines, Iowa, where he became a close friend of Governor Blaine who had run for Presidency. The children of their family included two boys who made enough through the personal manufacture of cigars to pay for night school training in law."

"One of their first cases in Des Moines was to defeat the State of Iowa in a Washington Supreme Court trial toward adopting Prohibition... A few years after the Chicago fire in 1871 the Blum family moved to Chicago to dwell in the well know Walnut Street locale near the lakefront."

"In 1888 I was born in the well known vicinity of Lincoln Park. I was the only child... My father acquired for the joint family interest four old buildings, without the ground, known as Erie Hotel. Therein for about a year my mother and I had resided when in 1898 a fire broke out resulting in the death of three guests. The soles of the feet of a young man friend were found on the street-car tracks, following his fall from the fifth floor window ledge of his room to his death."

"While my father was not a nervous person, being calm and collected as a rule, and my mother also was in no sense neurotic, I was appalled by the nervously excited state of various individuals following the fire. To be sure, the city newspapers made much of it. Accordingly when I was admitted to Northwestern University in 1907 it had become one of my purpsoes to investigate and knowledge of that day concerning the nature of nervousness and excited emotion and the treatment..."

"In 1909 I had completed the four year university course... I entered the graduate department of philosophy and psychology at Harvard in 1908 because Scott had referred to Professors William James, Josiah Royce and Hugo Muensterberg as "world record breakers". Notwithstanding their evident genius, I was severely disappointed because I failed to find in any of the three strictly scientific methodology... At the onset Professor Muensterberg had assigned to me a repetiton of the studies of Ranschberg entitled, "The Inhibition of Identicals" and had been greatly disappointed when I reported to him that my results were quite negative. It was evident also from the very outset that my methods in the laboratory were mathematically precise and free from bias.

"Upon personally investigating what was known of nervousness and excessive emotion in that era, I found to my amazement that these fields had been barren of investigation. Accordingly, after reading an account by the French psychologist, Fouillè, on "The Start of Surprise", I began my laboratory experiments with measurements of this involuntary reflex...

"One evening I was privileged to visit Professor William James, then reckoned by many as the world's greatest psychologist. My purpose was to seek information from him concerning an experimental inquiry into reflex nervous start. Although he had written on "The Gospel of Relaxation", having received so-called "training" by a Swedenborgian nurse, I found him an amazing spectacle of failure to relax. Conspicuously, he breathed irregularly, the tip of his beard was often in and out of his mouth, while his arms and legs fidgeted upon changing his position repeatedly. He turned to me, exclaiming impatiently, "Why don't you experimental psychologists study the whole man?"... I departed, feeling all the more that I must proceed in the laboratory entirely on my own judgement and methods.

"Quite different was my impression of Walter Cannon, then assistant professor of physiology at Harvard University. I found him the soul of precaution and precision in lecturing to his class, of which I had become a member... His modesty continued even after he had been granted the Nobel Prize. He visited me in my hotel offices in New York City for brief treatment as he expressed it, "in his declining years"..."

"My Ph.D. thesis was entitled: "Inhibition". It covered both physiological and psychological aspects. My popularity was low at ebb in Cambridge until an unexpected event entirely changed the picture. I was a member of the class in symbolic logic conducted by Professor Josiah Royce when the question of the nature of truth was brought up. Professor Royce quoted Pilot, 'What is truth?'. Evidently, like Pilot, Royce regarded the question as unanswerable or at least unanswered. To state this in the presence of a boy in his teens was perhaps too much! Accordingly I prepared a paper entitled, 'The Relational Account of Truth' and presented this as my term thesis. Professor Royce pronounced it a good paper and... told me to send it to the Journal of Philosophy, Psychology and Scientific Methods and to convey his approval.

"The appearance of the paper created a commotion of praises among the students... as well as among the professors... Although I was offered the highest rated fellowship of Harvard for...1910-11, I left Harvard for Cornell where I received an honorary fellowship without stipend. The lack of renumeration was painful, since it threw all financial burden directly upon my mother who supported herself and me as a court typist and stenographer, working beyond her strength. At Cornell I was disappointed with both Professor Titchener and the graduate students. Although both were drilled well in sensory psychology, I was amazed at their lack of training to observe what takes place internally during perception, understanding and thinking...

"In the fall of 1911, I entered medical school at the University of Chicago, but also became an assistant in the instruction of physiology to classes of medical students. My article entitled, 'Further Experiments on the Inhibition of Sensations' won for me an honor award in physiology...

"In the later years... I was appalled again at the complexity of the human organism in disease and disorder... Subsequently, during an internship at Cook County Hospital, the secondary only to the Wiener Krankenhaus, I had a unique opportunity to acquire diagnostic skill in internal medicine and also in organic neurology. In self-training during a most varied medical and surgical internship, I seemed to acquire skill in observation technique but also an ability to integrate my findings...Following my arrival in Chicago, in a conference with...Dr. Peter Bassoe, I informed him that...my chief purpose was scientific investigation. He replied that others had tried this but failed..."

"In 1925 I had been married happily to a youngster of 17 years, Elizabeth Ruth Silverman when I first saw her at my lectures. Although naive in matters of business, she had been brought up by her mother to devotion to the public interest. Our first child, Ruth Frances, was born in 1930. I had taught my wife technical relaxation during childbirth. Thus her labor was the first example of results in this field, years later to be popularized among obstetricians by Dr. Grantly Dick Reed... Two years later, the second child, Edmund Jr., was born, but this time delivered by the well-known Dr. William Dieckman, who had familiarized himself with labor under conditions of progressive relaxation...

"Years later (1949) Dr. F. J. Brown, professor of obstetrics at the University of London wrote: "Nothing has been more remarkable in the practice of obstetrics within the last ten years than the increasing appreciation of the value of principles enunciated by Edmund Jacobson in 1929 in his book "Progressive Relaxation" and afterward applied to midwifery by Grantly Dick Reed in his two books, "Natural Childbirth" and "Revelations of Childbirth."

"During subsequent years I devoted considerable personal time and attention to problems of national affairs. I met privately with General Groves in charge of army bomb weaponry (who cancelled a date with Gromiko to meet with me), with Admiral Blandy upon his return from Bikini following the use of the atom bomb there, and with Barney Baruch in New York concerning the Lilienthal Plan. These meetings were private and never publicized. Another interest in Washington was calling upon the successive doctors of each of the three presidents, Roosevelt, Eisenhower and Truman concerning the health of their important patients.

"In 1917 I introduced the low salt diet into medicine, but have never had occasion to employ it for my own health... In 1921, at the American Medical Association meeting, I introduced what was later to be christened "psychosomatic medicine"... In the early twenties I returned to the University of Chicago Department of Physiology. In 1925 I invited the department head, Professor

A. J. Carlson, to join me in research on the influence of relaxation upon the knee-jerk...Among the subjects to receive training in progressive relaxation was Arthur Steinhaus, later to become illustrious in the field of tension control and also the dean of George Williams College. At the University of Chicago from about 1924 to 1936 my investigations were aided by university funds but financed chiefly by my personal earnings in my Chicago and New York paractice of medicine.

"In 1927 I began the investigations which for the first time revealed the precise nature of mental activity as well as the measurement thereof in peripheral regions. The so-called relation of mind to body had been vague and philosophical... Thus, the nature of mental activities was removed from speculation whether they occur in parallel, in interaction or monistically with corresponding brain activity. In other words, for the first time in history the nature of mental activity became definitively established as a peripheral as well as a central (brain) phenomenon...Enclosed herewith ...you will find a photostat of a pamphlet I sent to every member of the American Congress...

"In my letter to these members, while the war was still in progress I suggested that the United Nations get together and form the World Peace Organization." It was subsequently that they joined to form what was at first called The United Nations Organization. In general this followed the departments I had previously suggested.

"It has been comforting to realize the honors graciously accorded to my measurements on the human mind by the directors of the 1977 Congress of Physiologists in Paris... "

"In your letter you mention the name of Professor Wigner whom I have not known personally but about whom I've heard much from a younger professor of theoretical physics. In the days of the development of the atom bomb I was kept fully informed of secret matters owing to my close association with Professor Walter Bartky who became the kingpin of such matters at the University of Chicago... I regret to write that Mrs. Fermi recently passed away. We met her often and intended to invite her to our apartment but never did so...

"Men with whom I have met or with whom I corresponded include: President Roosevelt and Governor Adams, who was in charge of foreign and many domestic policies during the Presidency of Dwight Eisenhower... Rear Admiral Morgan Watt became my patient and close friend from the time he was a Lieutenant Commander. He engineered the construction of the PT boats for D-Day in Europe. As I wrote you previously, it was he who invited no less than Admiral Nimitz to his home to meet me, which I considered ridiculous. Other outstanding men in the United States with whom I have been intimate include the famous Senator Douglas. In Washington I once gave a treatment to Governor Ribicoff of Connecticut, now senator, to illustrate the nature of progressive relaxation...

"Adler came over to see me personally. Professor Schultz, who belonged to the Hitler Guard, made the trip from Germany to visit me in Chicago on three different dates. You ask whom I know among painters. From time to time Beth and I have visited Anagoni (who is considered perhaps the foremost of all portrait painters) at his studio in Florence. He painted the portrait of Queen Elizabeth II of England and other members of the Royal Family. He also painted President Johnson."

"While visiting the Psychology Department at the University of Chicago, Aldous Huxley from England...came to our home for an evening... Both presidents of the Bell Telephone Laboratory, Oliver Buckley and Mervin Kelly, received training in progressive relaxation and were enthusiastic in their support and hopes that training in this field would become widespread in Europe as well as in America.

"My closest personal friends have included Oscar F. Mayer who had been a member of the lower German nobility as a forester in the Black Forest. His son, Oscar G. Mayer was my closest friend in high school, at Harvard and in Chicago until his death. He, Curt Holton of the Ethyl Corporation and I founded the Foundation for Scientific Relaxation in New York... Among other very close friends and pupils has been Rear Admiral Bart Hogan, Surgeon General of the United States Navy...

"President Roosevelt, along with our very close friend, Henry Pope, owner of the huge corporation which manufactured 'Bear Brand Hosiery', founded the Warm Springs Foundation. Both were interested in the disease, infantile paralysis. Henry Pope supplied all the money, however..."

"The greatest of all men in economics was Professor Irving Fisher. When nearing and passing the age of 80, he visited my clinic daily during one or two weeks each year... Greatly interested in what progressive relaxation could accomplish, he urged me to visit his former roomate, Secretary of State Dulles... On my subsequent visit to Washington, on his very busy day, the Surgeon General omitted luncheon in order to ask me questions regarding progressive relaxation on his own behalf. He stated that he had a skin disorder for which the following of the directions of my book, "You Must Relax" had been prescribed by his very famous skin specialist...

Some time later I got the photostat of a letter written after the 10th Annual Meeting of the Biofeedback Society of America last

February by Professor John D. Rugh which speaks for iteself:

"Dear Dr. Jacobson,

I am writing to thank you...Your presentation was truly the highlight of the meeting as indicated by the five minute standing ovation and by comments we received from the membership. The historical perspective and insight you presented were a learning experience for all of us. Your humorous remarks and personal anecdotes touched everyone's heart. The audience left with a feeling of warmth and respect for you and your wife. The contribution you have made to health science will not likely be surpassed; however, will be built upon by all of us attending the meeting. It was an honor to have you with us this year.

Sincerely yours, John D. Rugh, Ph.D."

Ladies and gentlemen, I hope that could give you an idea of what Edmund Jacobson's life was like and an impression of his person, by his own words and mine. In case you think that something was wrong you may be right insofar as one should not publish personal correspondence of persons living without their permission. But I am sure nobody could paint his life as well as Edmund Jacobson himself. He is not only a scientist but a fluent writer as well, and I hope he will agree with me and support me in this respect. I want to ask him to excuse me reminding him of the words of Shakespeare whom Edmund admires so much and who wrote in his Sonnet XXXV:

"No more be griev'd at that which thou hast done:
Roses have thorns, and silver foundtains mud;
Clouds and eclipses stain both men and sun,
And loathsome canker lives in sweetest bud."

I am well aware that my lecture is not perfect. Time is too short, and on the other hand I was too weak to drop details which are interesting to me.

Somerset Maugham, the famous writer and colleague, once said:

"Critics divide writers into those who have nothing to say and do not know how to say it, and those who know how to say it and have nothing to say".

It is up to you, ladies and gentlemen, to decide which group I belong to.

With this I am going to finish my lecture bearing in mind

Voltaire's warning:

"Woe to him who tells everything he knows!"

Thank you.

INDEX